Booby Traps

Booby Traps

A BOOK OF BRAS, BREASTS, AND BANDS

Maria Coffman, D.O.

Painted Turtle Press

Copyright © 2023 by Maria Coffman, D.O.

All rights reserved. No part of this book may be reproduced in any manner whatsoever without written permission except in the case of brief quotations embodied in critical articles and reviews.

United States of America
First Printing, 2023

ISBN 979-8-9872056-0-0
Library of Congress Control Number 2023916640
Cover design, illustrations, and interior photos by Maria Coffman, D.O.
Author's Photo by David Spencer, D.O.

Disclaimer
The information presented in this book is the author's opinion. It does not constitute health or medical advice. The content is for informational purposes only and is not intended to diagnose, treat, cure, or prevent any condition or disease.
Please seek advice from your physician for your personal health concerns prior to taking healthcare suggestions from this book.

For more information visit MariaCoffman.com

Disclaimer and Disclosure

Although Dr. Coffman is a licensed physician at the time of this writing, she is not your physician. Buying or reading this book does not form a physician-patient relationship. Any changes you choose to make or exercise you wish to try as presented in this book may affect your health and wellbeing. Seek advice from your physician for your personal health concerns prior to taking healthcare suggestions from this book.

Information presented in this book is the author's opinion. It does not constitute health or medical advice. The content is for informational purposes only and is not intended to diagnose, treat, cure, or prevent any condition or disease.

Wardrobe changes, lifestyle changes, exercises, and any other changes suggested or inspired by this book do not guarantee a specific outcome. For example, removing a bra for sleep does not guarantee your breasts will become larger, smaller, higher, or lower, or that you will sleep better or worse. No insights or suggestions should be construed as to guarantee a specific outcome. It is recommended that you consult with your physician for a plan to reach your specific health goals.

Although specific brands or products may be named in the book, these are given as examples or inspiration for your own research and do not constitute an endorsement on my part. I have not been offered nor accepted any money or gifts to endorse products.

This is a non-fiction work, but even so, some characters may be composites to lend reading clarity to the topic and to protect the privacy of any one individual.

Contents

Disclaimer and Disclosure — v
Dedication — ix

I
Underlayers

1. A Bra, by Any Other Name — 2
2. History of the Modern Brassiere — 5
3. Why We Wear Bras, and When We Don't! — 12
4. Bodies and Bras: The Match-up — 17
5. Bra (not) Fitting — 28
6. Measurements for Health — 32

II
Under it all

7. Anatomy: A New Perspective — 48
8. Anatomy Expanded: Form and Function — 55

III
Outfitting

9. Making the Most of What We Have — 90
10. What to Look For if Trying Something New — 98

11	Be Free! Thoughts on how to comfortably reduce or eliminate standard bra wearing	103
12	Tight Bands, No!	108
13	Breast Health and Self-care	112
14	Bras, Breasts, and Beyond: Engaging the Breast Appreciation Group	121

Appendix	123
References and Resources	125
Acknowledgements	129
About the Author	130

Dedicated to my mom, who first introduced me to breasts and bras.
"Why am I so plain and you're so fancy?"
observed her 4-year-old at bath time.

I

Underlayers

1

A Bra, by Any Other Name

I left my dorm room for a tai chi class in a mental fog under the cloud of an afternoon headache. An hour later I returned to clear bright skies and a renewed spirit. What had just happened? It was late summer during my freshman year of college in Kirksville, Missouri, and I was taking my first Tai Chi Chuan course with Master En Mow "John" Chiao. Through a sequence of movements and breath, Master Chiao had introduced our group of young Westerners to the concept of energy flow within and around the body. We were instructed to wear loose-fitting clothes to class, and Master Chiao would often respectfully tap a student's wrist if he saw a tight watch or elastic hairband on it. With short commands and an engaging smile, he conveyed, "Tight band, no!" followed by a dramatic inhalation. I followed his hands as they swept upward and out to float gently back to his sides. A serene smile lit his face and half-closed eyes until he spotted a belt. Belts were also a "no-no." We learned to arrive to class in bare feet, wearing loose sweatpants—hey, it was the '80s—and baggy T-shirts to let our energy flow freely. But no one mentioned our underwear. Apparently, the unseen cinched bands and shrinking undies—the fault of laundromat dryers I am sure, certainly no one gained weight freshman year!—were off-limits for discussion.

My health improved regularly with Tai Chi. Under the guidance of

Master Chiao's voice and waterfall gestures, I came to understand that circumferential bands on the body could impair the flow of the breath, the circulation, and an invisible energy field. I learned that removing them had an immediately-positive effect on one's health. I looked forward to our Tuesday and Thursday afternoon class, particularly because while I often arrived with a headache, rarely did I depart with one. I was intrigued and relieved. Subsequently, during medical school and postgraduate training, I discovered I could relieve many headaches simply by unhooking the back of my bra (folding the ends under discreetly) and loosening my belt. If a ponytail caused strain I unleashed my mane.

The first autumn during my osteopathic medical training at Kirksville College of Osteopathic Medicine I was studying images of the human heart, lungs, stomach, and intestines when Master Chiao's "Tight band. No!" came to mind. The initial images depicted the organs in their healthy natural state while a corresponding set displayed the disturbing effect of a woman's corset on organ position. Down the hall, a life-sized cardboard cut-out of a corseted woman stood in the school's museum. On one side, the photograph was overlaid with an image of the internal organs. It was similar to a "paper-doll" dressed-up but in reverse. The result revealed half of the woman's intestines squeezed into a position above the tightly cinched waist with the remainder pushed below the waistline. The liver and stomach were displaced upward, occupying precious lung space. They now impaired the descending motion of the diaphragm, rendering the fashionable corset wearer unable to take a full breath. Furthermore, the rearrangement of the organs left her prone to hypoxia and fainting. I thought about Master Chiao's circumferential bands. Women were led to believe that the narrow bands on modern bras were such an advancement over corsets. But were they? My failed attempts at a full breath while strapped inside mine indicated otherwise. Musing about the pretty young woman in the museum photo, I also wondered what was happening to the lymph vessels and veins draining her organs. I tried to imagine her arteries supplying nutrition and oxygen to her heart, lungs, and liver. I stalled in my thoughts. What oxygen? Could she even breathe? I unhooked my bra and walked away.

Fashion trends have squeezed throughout history, and meeting Doran Farnum, D.O., a legend in the field of osteopathic medicine, helped fill in a time gap for me. It was 2005, and we were attending an osteopathic manipulation workshop at Kirksville College of Osteopathic Medicine (KCOM), the founding school of osteopathy. My name tag read KCOM '95. Dr. Farnum's read KCOS, Kirksville School of Osteopathy '36. Was the year a typo? That should have been my first clue the fit physician might be older than he seemed. While he appeared to be a sassy septuagenarian, Dr. Farnum was actually 92 at the time and maintained an osteopathic practice in San Juan Capistrano, CA. Each year he returned to Kirksville for Founder's Day, and I was fortunate to become his lab partner for the workshops that year. During the lecture portion of one of the workshops, Dr. Melicien Tetambel, another remarkable D.O., reminded all of us to assess for the "bra-strap lesion"—a somatic dysfunction of the thoracic spine and ribs right along the bra band in most women. It's *that* common. The unassuming Dr. Farnum beside me giggled knowingly. I thought, "I bet he's felt a lot of bra band lesions, and girdles, over the decades. Probably even corsets!" Can you imagine? Decades, centuries later, and bra bands are still an issue. Darn, treating the spine and ribs affected by a bra band and continuing to wear the bra band won't fix the root cause. "Snap..."

2

History of the Modern Brassiere

By most accounts, the modern bra with its chest band, breast cups and shoulder straps owes its existence to a woman in the early 1800s who sewed two handkerchiefs together with a ribbon and pronounced women free from the corset. Mary Phelps Jacobs patented her designs in 1914. She would later change her given name and marry resulting in her more well-known name, Caresse Crosby, a literary giant. Fifteen years earlier, a French woman, Herminie Cadolle, had designed her corset-buster brassiere. These designs were meant to free women from the whalebone frames and tension-building lace-up closures of stays and corsets. And yet, more than a century later, remnants of these corsets and stays are still in place with wiring, boning, and shapers.

Modern history of the bra according to Dr. Coffman

I gave my perspective on the history of the modern bra to a colleague at a conference. Relating to the woman 25 years my junior, I realized I had a lot of experience in the evolution and social factors that shaped our bras in the past five decades. And with my mom and grandmothers, perhaps I could offer a good 70 years.

Granny panties, the classics, a good sturdy pair, inhabited the dresser drawers of Grandma "A." Nestled next to them were no-nonsense all-white polyester bras with Playtex cross-your-heart styling in the front. My other grandmother, Grandma "B," wore bras professionally fitted in the G-cup range. (Cup volume is all relative as you will see in later chapters.) These were by lingerie companies like Olga and Bali and came with an occasional embellishment, a lace applique perhaps, and were golden beige in color. Both variations of bras, the sturdy and the fancy, consisted of a single layer of non-stretch fabric with no lining and lots of seams. (It takes more than a few seams to turn a 2-dimensional piece of fabric into a geodesic dome.) The un-lined cups rumpled into wrinkles when laid on a flat surface. In the '70s it was rare to find underwire in bras with smaller cup sizes like AA, A, and B. Wires were reserved for larger cup sizes, C and greater. Padding was very uncommon. The majority of offerings were un-lined single layers of fabric with occasional options of "fiberfill-lined". Fiberfill is the fluffy white synthetic material you might see pop out of a sleeping bag after the dog helps you unpack from a camping trip. In grade school the old Sears catalog came to my friend's house each Christmas. After picking out our toy dream list, we would peek at the lingerie section. Matronly "foundations" in plain white, such a contrast from today's parade of prints, were displayed modestly on the models. I recall very few underwire styles and only two or three color options, namely, white, beige, and black. The minimizer bra section was equally curious. "What's a minimizer?" we wondered. And, "Why?" Were we supposed to have them or hide them? These questions began and never really stopped.

A 1970s everyday bra was made of non-stretch, woven fabric, lots of seams, with little to no decoration, and was usually unlined. A lined bra was just that, a second layer of fabric. Padded bras were reserved for costumes, dress-up or formal wear. Adults said they were easy to spot and not desirable: "Don't stuff your bra or it will look fake and obvious." But, lacking padding, visible nipple show-through was a problem. Girls piled on extra sweaters to cover up on cold days and were told to cross their arms over their chest, hold a book in front, do whatever was needed to keep their nipples from showing.

The '80s came along, and Lycra/Spandex entered the lingerie arena. Suddenly everything soft, breast tissue included, began to feel tense like a trampoline. Single-frame cartoons joked of women in locker rooms exploding out of shiny tights and leotards after aerobic dance classes. I would later learn of the chronic change in subcutaneous tissue texture from a soft silky substance to "Knox Blocks Jell-O" stiffness in patients who wore spandex shapers on a daily basis. Science class tells us that substances exist in three states: gas, liquid and solid. The molecules of a gas are the farthest apart and those in solids are tightly packed. Molecules of gas can be compressed into a liquid and liquids can be compressed into a solid. Carbon dioxide fits this model. It is one of the gases we breathe in the air. It can be compressed into liquid and finally, with enough spandex, oops, enough pressure, it can become a solid, "dry ice" for making theater-effect fog roll out from a cooler.

Hard bodies and the super-thin were not enough to keep our interest. The '90s burst onto the scene and with it the blockbuster marketing of WonderBra. These new designs produced cleavage where demure chests had been before. Abundant and strategic push-up padding, wiring, side-stays, and the rib-snug band really made them "pop." Women were back in the workforce and ready to climb corporate ladders. Pantsuits, skirt suits, and business attire (but with a distinctively female—not to be confused with "feminine"—edge) were the rage. Enter WonderBra's famed photo and one-line ad: Leaping across the back cover of *Vogue* magazine, a blond bombshell sported a business-style pantsuit minus the shirt. Her tiger expression and "got it all" look showcased her breasts encased in WonderBra. It read, "If men had 'em they'd wear WonderBra every day." The implied messages were that 1. Men weren't holding back their fancy underwear for "special occasions." 2. Push-up bras weren't just for costumes and formal occasions anymore and 3. Women could use their cleavage to climb the corporate ladder.

Next up, Victoria's Secret. Need I say more? I do. I credit the T-shirt bra and its marketing to Victoria's Secret. Where WonderBra took us up and over the top, Victoria's Secret "Body by Victoria" line launched in the late '90s marketing "natural" sex appeal. A "faux" naturalness, to be sure, promising an ideal of what we could look and feel like with a "perfect" body. This is the premise of the T-shirt bra: to give a "natural" seamless profile without nipples. Victoria's Secret's celebrated "angels" gave us select options. The catalog displayed intimates on proportionately large bosom-to-body volumes and domed breast shapes. I do not know if this was just the bras. I suspect a duct tape trick, silicone cutlets, make-up magic or a combination to achieve the effect. Mainstream and marketing's ideal breast shape mirrored a mall mannequin, nipple-free half honeydews.

With fashion becoming more and more casual even in the workplace and shirt fabrics shifting from starched wovens to clingy knits, the T-shirt bra provided relief for nipple camouflage and really filled a gap in bra coverage. A full cup of polyurethane foam padding and an underwire frame, this bra's cup shape did not flatten out on the floor. Instead they sat up like little Baked Alaska merengue cakes. The first time I saw one in a laundry basket, I thought of how embarrassed my friends and I would have been in middle school, or even college, for someone to see our bras sitting up as though breasts were still in it. Bra fashion and acceptance had definitely come a long way.

Viewing the decades of bra trends as a theater stage, the foam cups part as the "corps de ballet" leaps center stage sporting—"tah-da!"—the JogBra. The grandmother of all sports bras was developed in the 1980's by runner Lisa Lindahl and inspired by her husband's athletic drawer. The JogBra (first called the Jock Bra owing to its origins—now you know) filled another gap of the 1980s and '90s. Title IX had opened up sports to women but what were we to wear? The JogBra solution was born from Adam's rib, or someplace nearby. Actually, it was two jock straps sewn together. From the sports bra's humble beginnings in combination with '80's charismatic performer, Madonna, ensuring underwear was outerwear, the sports bra came out front and center, and remained there. Daily variations include yoga tops, no shirt required; compression equipment (take it off as soon as possible, doctor's orders); and the comfort bra, now a model offered by nearly every bra-maker.

A new millennia and the internet brought the next evolution in breast coverage. Buy a bra online? Yep, just like shoes online. Preposterous. Everyone knows bras and shoes need to be properly fitted in person! Yes, but companies take that into account by offering free returns. With brick and mortar out of the picture, there's more room for enticing web pages full of colors, lace and creativity. Video reviews of regular people with regular bodies ready to "share" enhance the shopping experience. I am still moved by the woman who posted on a semi-secure site her review of an adhesive "bra". These creations have come a long way from Band-Aids as nipple covers. Sticky bras are now touted to lift and shape any breast size. The video blogger's breast volume was close to 70 ounces (2 liters) per breast. Alas, the adhesive lift failed miserably. I add "miserably" due to the ending footage of the video when she attempted to peel the patches from her nipple as her audience cringed.

On a better note, in recent years I've witnessed a conscious movement of returning to natural fibers—organic cotton, wool, linen and bamboo. I've also seen the classic underwire T-shirt bra give way to an even smoother silhouette sans wire. True Body, in True&Co.'s online-only store is an example. Cross-overs and combinations of structured fashion and fitness bras abound in nearly every color, fabric, design and size. The challenge remains, however, to find one that embodies all of these characteristics. Can you imagine a soft texture, heart-healthy fit *and* non-toxic materials?

Bras abroad

Through my osteopathic career I have been given a wonderful network of girlfriends and colleagues around the globe. Among our various topics of girl talk have been discussions about the custom of bra wearing and social expectations. I asked some of them whether they would quiz their mothers and grandmothers about the custom for as far back as they recalled. The responses surprised me. It seems that wearing bras is ubiquitous around the globe! Even more surprising to me was the uniform understanding that any hint of nipples is a "no-no" in polite company. Friends interviewing their mothers and grandmothers affirmed that this has been the case for at least two generations in the U.S. and in places like Africa, India, South America and Australia. Read on for snippets of our conversations by locale.

Nigeria: Everyone wears a bra, starting at puberty. If you cannot afford to buy one, you go to the local tailor, who will make one for you.

India: An American family member was attending a wedding in Southern India in traditional dress. The bodice of her sari seemed to fit like a bra, so she inquired if one was necessary under it. "Oh yes!" replied her Indian host.

Rural India of the 1960's was a more varied story. My father-in-law recalls seeing all levels of breast coverage while riding public busses during his Peace Corps days. Less wealth correlated to less coverage. More affluence meant more coverage.

Chile and Argentina: My well-traveled colleague relates that noticeable nipples are an issue everywhere she has journeyed—in the northern and southern hemispheres, and throughout the east and the west. Her experience at her second home in Argentina mirrored mine during a visit to coastal Chile. The dress code is similar to ours in North America. Laid-back beach scenes coexist with covered and modest town time.

China: A Northern Chinese friend described something of a halter top worn under traditional clothing. A piece of cloth covers the front and is held in place with a tie behind the neck and one around the waist.

"Certainly, there still has to be a place on Earth where the bra has not dominated," I thought.

I have to admit, my childhood view of global culture was strongly influenced by *National Geographic* magazine. People of remote tribes featured on those pages did not wear shirts or much else whether they were male or female. Decades later, I pondered the existence and location of these bra-free people.

"Turkana."

"Turkana?" I echoed in question.

My Kenyan friend's proper British accent rang clearly across our internet call, "In the southern part of Kenya, they still wear very little there. No, no shirts, nor pants. The men sometimes wear a little flap over their thingy." She said it with a straight face.

Naturally, I immediately googled the tip. And after a moment of stunned shock (no, not from nudity) I doubled into laughter. The news article that popped up featured a Kenyan singer native to Turkana who had returned home for a community fundraiser. The richly colored photographs featured local dancers with the beautiful celebrity leading them, barefoot, clad in a traditional woven, beaded skirt and a *bra*. It wasn't just any bra; this was a sparkling orange confection, sequined and underwired, like fresh tropical fruit. Although my friend assured me that the photo was just for publicity, my braless assumptions were shattered. It *is* a small world, after all, and the bra has it covered.

Through my own travels I have experienced differing levels of bra/breast coverage customs. The divisions of time and place can seem surreal. Expectations at a specific locale today can be entirely different tomorrow. Imagine a festival at a downtown park, perhaps anything goes! But, come Monday morning one had better button –up! Regions shift, too, over time. For example, during a delightful chilly dip in Lake Zurich one summer day in 2015 while I was visiting family friends, some of the women swam only in bikini bottoms. Interestingly, it was only the older women who did this. Topless bathing seemed tolerated but not really encouraged at that time and location—unlike the Portuguese beach I visited in 1993, where it seemed more the norm. But regardless of country or decade, tops were back in place within two meters of the lake shore or beach edge.

Coverage expectations are dependent on all kinds of factors, not the least of which is location. Perhaps an Australian comic strip of a man at a beach, wearing nothing but racing briefs, shows it best: The opening frame depicts him walking along the water's edge. Subsequent frames have him striding across the beach (still clothed only in spandex swimwear), up a set of steps, down a sidewalk, across a street, and finally arriving at a cafe. The caption simply reads: "Speedos, Speedos, Speedos, undies, undies, undies."

3

Why We Wear Bras, and When We Don't!

In my practice many women have shared their bra stories and solutions with me. Osteopathy is based on the body's innate ability to heal when obstacles are removed, and sometimes that is the bra band. I am always relieved to be able to treat a patient who arrives sans le brassiere. While I am hesitant to ask whether "bra-free" is an everyday occurrence or just for the appointment, a few patients answer my silent question.

"I don't wear one," announces an 80-year-old retired biologist as she pulls out the hem of her undershirt to show-and-tell her solution. A slender patient in her 50s prefers a tank top undershirt and a loose overshirt. A full-breasted homeschooling mother of three says, "They aren't healthy. I just wear things so you can't tell—looser tops and prints."

College students, gardeners, and professionals have been among my patients who dress bra-free (though usually under the radar).

So, why *do* we wear them?

We wear them for the same reasons we don't!

Comfort

The physical discomfort experienced by some women during high impact exercise can be decreased with a bracing bra—a well-fitted sports bra worn for that activity only. Others tell me that sweat or dampness under their breasts is less uncomfortable with a bra on or with their breasts lifted up. My preference for padded cups—a.k.a. a breast plate for impact protection—came about while raising small rugby players at home. ("Mommy! Catch!" shrieked my toddler as he flung himself from the tabletop toward my unsuspecting chest.)

Custom and culture

We saw the pervasive custom of bra wearing in the previous chapter. What drives these customs?

Cultural notions of modesty and attention, both desired and undesired, are the point of bras in public. What a woman would choose to wear or not wear, just for her, is shifted when in public. On her own, a woman often prefers comfort and function. Aesthetics are icing on the cake. By aesthetics I am referring to both how she likes the styling of her undergarments—lacy or minimalist—and how she wants to look in her clothes whether she wears one or not.

A woman considers her "look" and how she will be perceived in a given setting. Is it a professional setting or a casual beach event with friends? Does she want to blend in or stand out? Social media posts allude to the dual messages sent to women: "Look sexy, and don't get killed." As women, we select our bras to provide a measure of physical comfort, coverage, and/or a particular physical shape, all the while, knowingly or not we are influenced by our culture. Our age, socio-economics, our families and our communities, both local and extended, all play a part in shaping our clothing choices.

All humans have biases. If you feel aware of your biases that is amazing and probably no longer fits the definition of a true bias, meaning one that is unknown. A true bias shows up when you look around flabbergasted because "it" (whatever disruption "it" may be) is SO obvious, but not to whomever it is that stoked the emotion.

I once was crossing the street from a business area to a park in Missouri with a lake on the other side. The lake included a swimming beach that was quite popular with families in the summer. At the busy crosswalk, beachgoers exited the park and others entered, some in beachwear but most dressed for walking. There I witnessed a clashing of public-attire expectations. Headed toward me, in a typical chaotic frenzy of tired children, was a young family of five. Their loose, long hair gave off a beachy boho vibe with a heavy dose of hippie. Under the woman's left arm nestled a naked infant clinging to his mother's bare breast like a monkey. The mother's free hand held that of a tousled-hair toddler, and her right breast covered the remainder of her torso. Between the blowing hair, kids, bags and crowded walkway, it took me a moment to register the shirtlessness. I did, though, just like everyone else.

"FINALLY!" I thought.

My mind jumped to the 1989 New York law that had made it legal for women to be topless in public. I diverted my gaze toward the lake. Then a strange choking sound behind me caught my attention. I turned to see a middle-aged couple staring at the half-clothed family. The woman attempted to remain poised as her male partner gasped, choked back words, and turned beet red. He shook and pointed vigorously at the exposed skin. The crowd's attention was shifted to him as we continued toward the lake away from the unaware family.

Getting back to the idea of bias, when we have a solid belief that we hold as a truth (in this case, that breasts and bottoms should be covered while in public) and someone is "breaking" it with their own beliefs, we feel uncomfortable. Wronged even. This is bias. Culture, media, and marketing use biases as tools to their advantage. Marketers play to our biases to sell products and services. Marketing reflects our perceptions of success, affluence, humility, beauty, modesty, and norm-breaking. But it also shapes them. It works both ways. Marketing begins by selling a solution to a problem and in so doing often creates the perception of a problem. These perceptions underlie our future choices and define our societal norms.

Fear

Emotions are powerful motivators. Fear is one of the most potent. Provoke just enough fear to get a predictable response (but just short of a flight, fight or freeze one), and you have control.

What fear keeps bras on? Fear of sagging. Nobody really wants to feel vain about their breast shape, but "Won't they droop if I don't wear a bra?" is a common concern. Our culture makes us feel discomfort with our bodies—and our breasts—changing shape as we get older. Many people experience feelings of sadness or loss when confronted with these changes, especially if the change is looked down upon by society.

Like any tool, a bra can be useful or a hindrance. Women wear them to be comfortable physically or socially and don't wear them for the same reasons. For each patient who told me they wore a bra to help with back pain, another said they took it off to relieve discomfort. And for each who said their breasts hurt too much to go braless, another found their breast congestion and pain subsided dramatically after being bra-free.

By far, the biggest reason women choose to go without a bra is the challenge of finding one that fits. Here is where this book can make the biggest impact. Regardless of any details and research cited here, this is the big empowering secret: *There are no standard sizes.*

There is no gold standard for measuring a person for a bra. There is no single measurement of a consistent bra fit even among bras labeled with the same band and cup. A 36C by two different designers, or a 36C in two different styles in the same brand, will hold different volumes of breast tissue and have different lengths in the actual band. Even if how to measure the body and how to calculate a "size" were standardized, the actual product, the bra, is not.

For that reason, I give you the go-ahead to toss out your measuring tape. Measure your body with an unmarked string. Removing the numerical data lets your right and left brain work together for an even better interpretation and decision-making process. It even reduces potential anxiety in the measuring process. "Do I measure up?" No matter! Place the string around the space you want the bra to cover—first, the ribcage and then the bust line. Mark the string at the point where the string completes its circle around your body. Next, take your string and measure the band and bust lengths of some bra choices. See which bras match up with *your* measurements.

Note: They may never match up. Keep reading!

4

Bodies and Bras: The Match-up

"Why doesn't your little girl run as fast as the boys anymore?"

For the fourth year in a row, I was watching runners at my children's elementary school Spring Field Day. Previous years had seen a girl win the mile race with an even mix of boys and girls finishing in the top ten. This year the girls began to fade early—and I would witness it again next year. What had changed? Boys' testosterone and muscle mass do matter. But a spike in testosterone production for boys takes place during middle school, around ages 11–13. These were 8-year-olds. What else was contributing to the sudden differences in speed? Tell-tale dents tugging under the T-shirts of the prepubescent girls revealed the source. Breasts or not, these little ones were wearing compression sportsbras. For most of them, there was nothing to be compressed except their breathing capacity which explained the winded gasps as they crossed the finish line. Despite this disadvantage my own daughter wanted one for gym class. The girls were required to change clothes for P.E. and no one wanted to be naked while others sported bras. Hence, our first mother-daughter bra-shopping adventure began much earlier than anticipated.

As an osteopathic physician my hands had felt the locked-up function of patient's tissues with tight-fitting clothes. And, as a grown woman I knew the difficulties women faced searching for a physiologically compatible piece of underwear. But wow, I was not prepared for the children's bra section of our local store. Our first bra hunt was a fast-paced world away from the "foundations" department and professional fitters I had experienced with my mom. Pull-over bras labeled XS through XL were doll sized! Somehow my eight-year-old agreed to the one that fit comfortably, an"XL", on her 48-pound frame. I promised to remove the tag at home. She went on to enjoy track and field competing in the mile event in middle school and high school, rarely finishing out of breath. How many other girls would have continued to run if they had been able to breathe easily? If they knew the balance between bounce and breath?

In this chapter we will apply our math sense to see what adds up and what does not in an effort to find that "balance point".

Breast gland shape vs. bra cup shape

Breast tissue's actual shape is similar to an apostrophe. It does not form circular discs or domes, but actually has a tail extending toward the axilla (armpit).

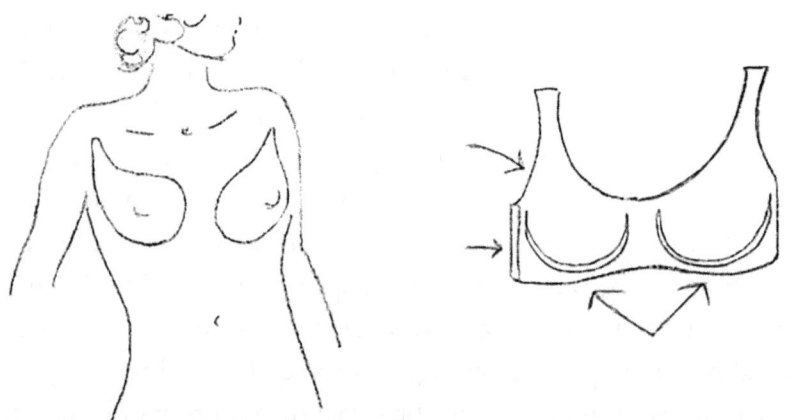

Figure 4.1: Breast Gland Shape and Bra Cup Shape
Left shows tear-drop shape and placement of breast gland. On the right a common bra style reveals cups defined by a C-shaped wire, armhole edges with pressure to the tail of the breast, and boning or stays to the side of the cups.

Breast tissue has a shape like an apostrophe, circular but with a tail. Bra cups don't have tails. The body and bra don't match.

Conclusion: Bra cups are not shaped like breasts.

Ribcage shape vs. bra band shape

A ribcage has sides. It has three-dimensional depth to provide structure and protection for internal organs such as heart, lungs and blood vessels.

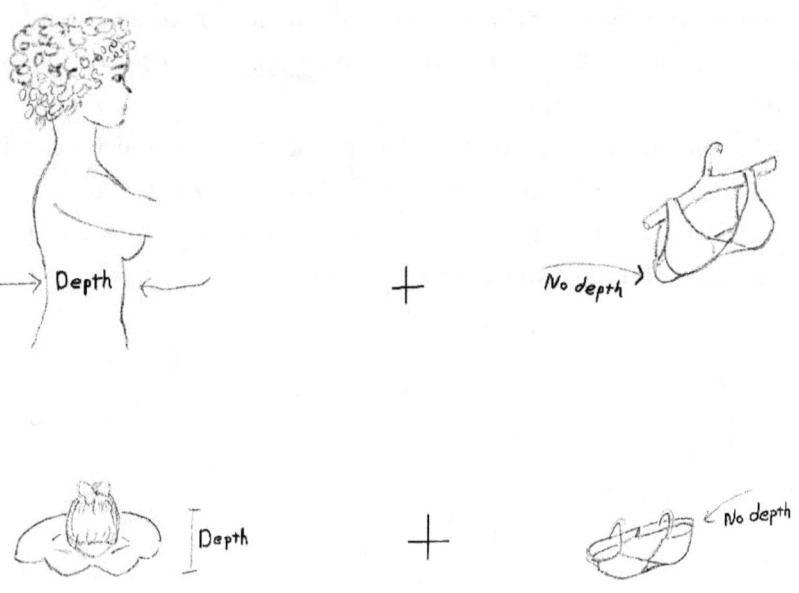

Figure 4.2: Side View and Bird's Eye View of Ribcage and Bra
Bras don't have sides. There is no depth. A ribcage has depth for organs. The body and bra don't match.

Conclusion: Bra bands are not shaped like a human ribcage.
Corollary: Semi-circle cups + lack of sides on bands = uh-oh.

Shoulders vs. straps

Using the analogy of an ankle sprain I will share insight on braces. A brace is something that straps on, cinches down, and holds part of you in one position until it is removed. Knee brace, ankle brace, breast brace. A bra. Exactly. A less immobilizing brace is an "Ace." Not really, that's just one brand that has become synonymous with elastic bandages. Ace wraps on an ankle, knee or chest (compression bras) have similar effects as a full brace. For mild to moderate sprains patients are instructed to remove a brace or wrap as often as possible, ideally every hour or more when at rest and to elevate the area for lymph drainage. When they are ready to go back to activities I recommend applying the brace or ace during activity and removing it afterward. Ankles, knees, and breasts all need circulation. All types of circulation are needed: energetic, lymph, blood, and neurotransmitters.

Shoulder tops are naturally smooth and sometimes defined with muscle. But they lack notches for straps. Atrophied grooves form under chronic pressure such as undersized bras on growing girls or years of narrow, tension-loaded straps on women.

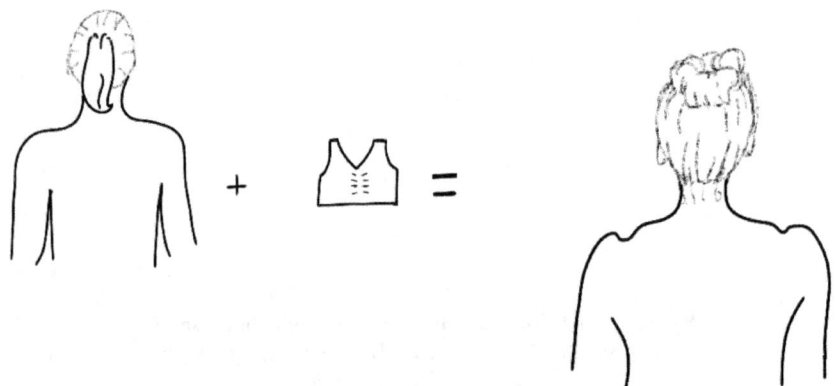

Figure 4.3: Shoulder Tops vs Shoulder Straps
A. Child's smooth shoulder. B. Pressure straps on bras. C. Grooved shoulder with subcutaneous fat atrophy due to chronic pressure.

Conclusion: Tension- loaded straps cause grooves through pressure necrosis.

Light-absorbing skin vs. light-blocking fabric

Have you ever felt yourself glowing with happiness, expectation, and fulfillment? Would you believe you actually were glowing? Yes, you! Your radiant self emits photons, minute particles of light. In a process of bioluminescence we all glow, but we glow brighter when we are fully charged. Humans also require full spectrum light for cellular processes such as the pathway converting pro-vitamin D3 to the active form used in tissues. Other parts of the visible light spectrum synchronize our pineal gland in the brain to schedule our daily physiologic cycle. Nature permits perky hormones like cortisol to increase during daytime hours and sedating sleepy ones like melatonin to increase for night time. In an osteopathic course from Australia I was introduced to the effects of light and sound frequency on red blood cells. The concept is that with each heartbeat the red blood cells passing through the heart and lungs are programmed with light and sound for their next mission out to tissue. Amazing! Our bodies both emit and absorb light photons.

Returning to the bra-to-body match-up, we find current day bras are darn near lightproof! I was inspired to share this observation after noticing a fair-skinned gardener's upper back at the end of summer season. During outdoor work she had worn long-sleeved, sun-protective clothing over a loose racerback bra. She also avoided sun between the hours of 10 a.m. and 2 p.m. Despite these precautions and a tendency not to tan, there was a distinct ivory imprint of racerback bra between her shoulder blades. Naturally, I inquired. The bra had one layer of cotton and polyester knit for the back and two layers in front. She had removed the optional foam cup inserts for work.

The scene set me thinking of how often our "fronts," or breasts, may have access to light through a layer or two of cloth. Modern bras have two layers of cloth with 2 to 8 mm of dense foam cups. Let the idea of skin access to light pique your interest. There is more information coming forward on light therapy as a healing modality. Future studies will show the benefits and risks of full spectrum, native, and non-native sources of light helping to shape our healthy choices in clothing.

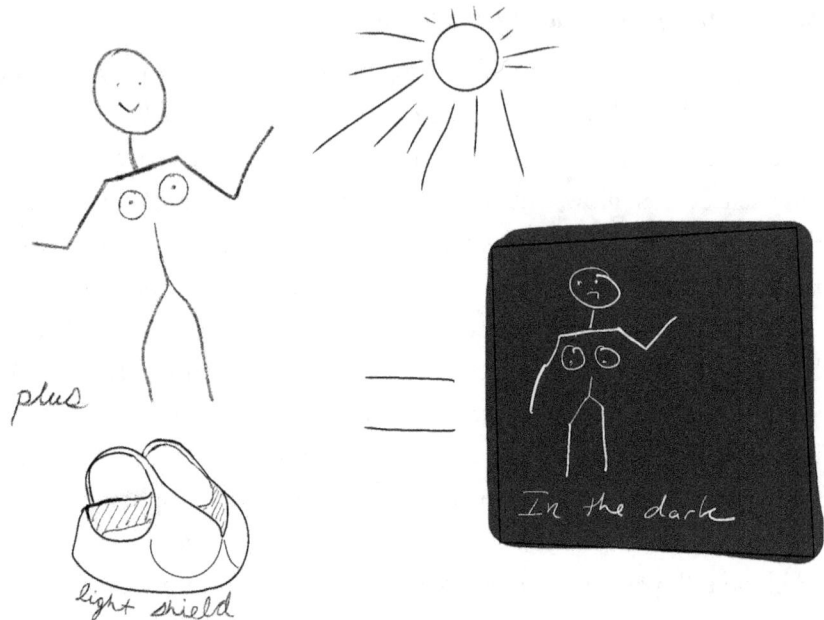

Figure 4.4: In the Dark
Living tissue needs light for biochemical reactions. Layers of cloth and padding selectively block or filter light.

Conclusion: Most bras block all light to our skin and tissues and to what extent this affects breasts is still unknown. We'll keep an open mind as we learn more about our own bioluminescence and effects of different types of light exposure on tissue health.

Self-regulating temperature vs. self-heating elements

Optimal biochemical reactions occur at specific temperatures. In general, chemical reactions are accelerated with increased temperature and slowed with lower temperature. Enzymatic action, methylation, building, and breaking down all have a proper rate to keep cell life in balance. The human body with its infinite wisdom continually scans and maintains proper temperature for tissues. As mammals, we maintain our own internal temperature, not the environment's temperature. When we insulate breasts with padding and foam then isolate those parts with wires and bands the auto-regulation of breast temperature is really challenged!

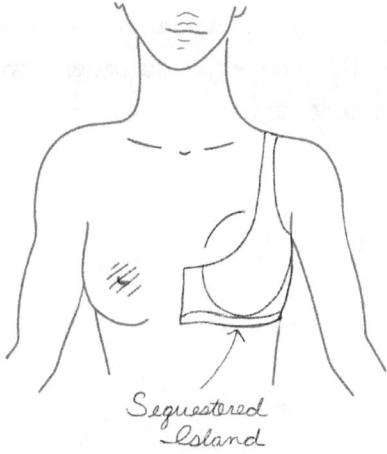

Figure 4.5: Sequestered Islands
Padded, insulated cups compress, heat and isolate the breast tissue creating sequestered islands. The islands are cut-off from the mainland highways of blood and lymph, from fresh nutrients, hormonal temperature regulation and cellular drainage of cellular debris.

Conclusion: Insulated bra cups + breasts in cups = heated breast cells.

Subtle energy flow vs. obvious obstructions

The human body has a complex system of electrical and subtle energy. Osteopathy describes neurolymphatic points known as Chapman's Reflexes on the surface of the body. These energy centers on the surface correlate to internal organs and can be used to diagnose and treat dysfunction. Several are located along the line just under the bottom edge of a bra band and cup. Most of these neurolymphatic locations are quite tender to touch related to congestion.

Acupuncture points along meridians in traditional Chinese medicine are also present throughout the torso. Liver, spleen, and pericardium meridians flow around and under each breast. Twelve pairs of major meridians all pass through the torso. Donna Eden of Energy Medicine fame relates her vision of shoulder bag or backpack straps cutting through multiple meridians as they traverse a shoulder. She sees the natural crossover pattern of energy being disrupted. A homolateral pattern results, associated with fatigue and depression, due to an inability to recharge one's battery. I sense the same effect on patients wearing "frontpacks", bust holders, with shoulder straps.

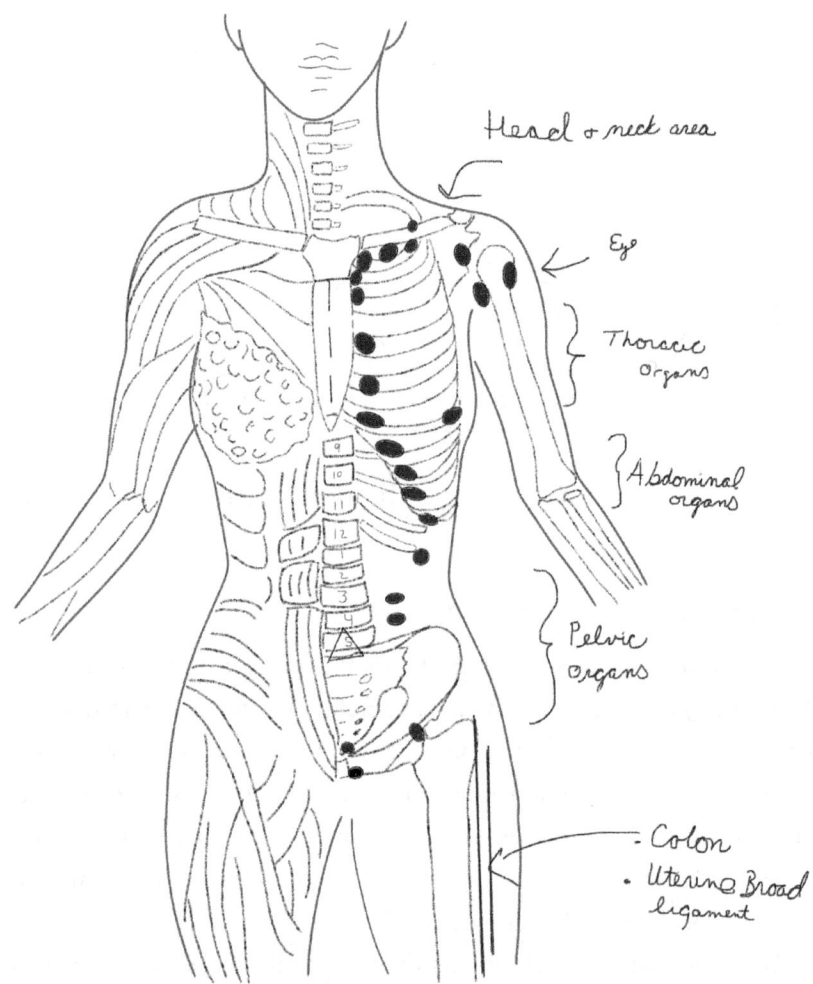

Figure 4.6: Chapman's Reflex Points Summary
The blackened ovals and lines represent reflex points on the surface of the body related to inside parts such as sinuses, retina, heart, lungs, and abdominal-pelvic organs. They exist on the right and left sides of the body mirror-image. A few are specific to their side such as appendix. Shoulder-straps, bands, wires, and hooks are visible obstructions to the invisible energy flow connecting body and organs.

Chapman's Reflex Points, also called neurolymphatic points, are both diagnostic and therapeutic. Tissue texture changes or tenderness over a point can indicate dysfunction in the related organ. Massaging or tapping a point can help clear congestion of the reflex point and its associated organ. Many of the organ reflexes are on the ribcage as shown and are affected by chronic pressure of clothing.

Conclusion: Bras are not designed for energy flow either.

Self-regulating detoxification and repair vs. chemical and electromagnetic field exposure

This section is a little different as we lump two sources of toxins together, non-native EMFs and chemical exposures. The end result of any toxic encounter is a detoxification of the tissue and repair of the remaining cells. Toxins of every source add up so it's important to reduce exposures of all types and to support the detoxification process.

Electromagnetic fields, native and non-native, have come to the forefront of integrative health. These non-visible fields are produced from things like electrical wiring in homes (assuming the breaker is on). Magnetic fields are produced by electrical motors: Your blender or a fan when turned on is an example. The newest and hugest increase in EMFs comes from radiofrequencies. Anything used to transmit information through air is in this higher frequency group. Wi-Fi, baby monitors, cordless phones, cellular phones, and microwave ovens are everyday examples. In healthcare, many types of frequency fields are used to image the body such as x-rays and ultrasound. Wireless devices such as heart rhythm monitors and continuous glucose monitors are also used to transmit information to or from a patient.

Focusing on the first one—electrical fields—and its relationship to lingerie is quite illuminating. Do you recall lightning rods atop tall buildings and barns? They are metal rods. Since metal attracts electrical fields it is an "antenna"—just like underwire in a brassiere. Antennae attract an electrical field and amplify it, potentiating the frequency. Metal in the body, primarily iron in red blood cells oscillates with this alternating current 60 times a second for U.S. electrical system of 60 Hz.

Conclusion: Underwire antennae in the presence of household electrical fields lead to disturbances in function of red blood cells and other tissues.

We are exposed to chemicals all around us, in our air, water, food, and clothing. Absorption of potentially harmful chemicals depends on several factors, including amounts of the chemicals and how long someone is in contact with them. Another important factor is the type of tissue in contact. Vapors that are inhaled through nasal openings into lungs are readily absorbed into the body as are chemicals ingested through the mouth to stomach. Skin is able to absorb toxins as well. Thick, dry skin (e.g., calloused feet) absorbs least whereas thin, highly vascular skin (underarms and groin) absorbs most.

Breasts have several high absorption properties: thin delicate skin, good vascularization, and doors. Doors? Yes, well, pores actually. Mammary papillae aka "nipples" are the end of milk ducts and hence there are little pores for milk to come out and little doors for chemicals to go in. Medical studies show promise in administering chemotherapy agents directly to breast tissue, especially the ductal system, through these papillae.

So, what else is absorbed into the breast via the ducts? Topical creams and lotions, and chemical vapors. One up close source of vapors is padding in bra cups. Polyurethane foam and memory foam can outgas for the life of the foam no matter how many times it is washed. New fabrics and garments are fumigated with pesticides for shipping. Even natural fibers such as cotton and linen are grown with multiple chemical crop sprays unless specifically produced organically. OKEO-Tex is an organization setting standards for reduced toxins in textiles. Look for OEKO-Tex 100 ratings on garment labels for fabric free of 100 known toxins.

Absorption of toxins in lingerie textiles through papillae leads to chemical toxins inside breast ducts.

Given the inevitability that our skin and mammary papillae will have contact with a toxin at some point, what is a cell to do? De-toxify of course. Lymph to the rescue! That sounds so dramatic, like an emergency, but this is actually part of moment-to-moment homeostasis in a cell's life. Taking trash out, recycling, and releasing are part of the living process. Tissues are designed with lymphatic pathways to collect and transport interstitial fluid for cleaning in lymph nodes, spleen, liver, and kidneys. Skin is special, too; its detoxification methods are to simply "sweat and slough"!

Difficulties arise when we preferentially sequester certain parts and then tie off those parts with compression from the rest of the body.

Conclusions: Absorption of toxins in lingerie textiles through papillae leads to chemical toxins inside breast ducts. And,

Tight clothing leads to impaired drainage of lymph and toxins.

In this chapter, we have explored with some humor ways in which various bras may be compromising to your body. While it takes some intrigue out of lingerie, this is what we need as we look at Chapter 5, "Bra *(not)* Fitting." These insights can help you choose the best bra or braless option for a given situation.

5

Bra (not) Fitting

So, you've uncovered the mismatch between bras and bodies and you want to explore more. In chapters 5 and 6 we look at the background of bra-fitting and women's perceptions about fitting. We will explore the various measurements and establish a basis for tossing the tape in favor of what you actually see and feel. Along the way you will find a stream of wisdom filling the space of health and breath.

Is everyone hard to fit or is it the bra?

When asked about their bras the most frequent feeling a women expresses is that she has a particular abnormality that makes her bra fitting situation unusually difficult. It sounds something like this:

I have a big ribcage so I'm hard to fit.

I have a small ribcage so it's hard to fit.

I gained weight, now I'm hard to fit.

I lost weight, nothing fits. I'm tall, the straps don't fit. I'm short, the straps don't fit.

I have a broad back, I have broad shoulders, I have narrow shoulders. I'm pregnant, I'm breastfeeding, I breastfed. My breasts are too big, my breasts are small, and they are uneven. I had augmentation, I had a reduction. I had a mastectomy. I had reconstruction. I had radiation. I have tender scar tissue.

My bras are fine, I'm just fat.

I remember a day growing up feeling particularly overwhelmed. My dad said "If *everything* around you is a problem, the problem might be *you*." Hmm. If *all women* are hard to fit in a bra, the problem might be *the bra*!

What I really hear with the litany of special and unique challenges for women is that women and bras are not a good match most of the time. Why? Humans are alive. Our bodies are in a continual state of change and balance to maintain homeostasis. Moment by moment are changes in physical form; bending left and right, changes in composition; more or less water, protein or fat, and changes in volume or size. I have seen some impressive bras, but they pale in comparison to an amazing human.

The question remains, was anyone comfy in their bra? Years ago a dear friend said "My bras are so comfortable, I sleep in them" That was 25 years ago. I'll give her a call to check up… The giggles start as I recount our morning conversation over cardamom coffee. "Did I say that? Oh! I don't sleep in them anymore. Not for a long time. Hmm, yes, a longtime."

Persevering, I found a bra match-up success story amidst the dismay. Another friend shared her recent happy bra story with me. She used a bra size calculator online to measure and auto-calculate a suggested size. She then ordered a U.K.-sized bra. It is said that the U.K. has standardized their bra sizing by government mandate. My friend related that it was the first time in 40 years of bra wearing that she didn't try to rip it off coming in the front door after work. She, like so many women, was certain she was "hard to fit." A petite height, extra curves, and generous cup size with prior surgical scars to avoid irritating, I agreed there were challenges. Finding a bra that kept her comfortable was a notable achievement. But, it had underwire, darn it. So, please don't sleep in it.

Inspired by her success we measured and calculated my size using on-line tools suggested on Reddit as well. I ordered from a different UK company to find something wire-free and received a matronly bra in its 2 "equivalent sizes." One was a 34-inch band, the other 32. The 34 fit just like the company's video of a perfect fitting. On the middle hook there were no back or underarm bulges of skin. The gore, the fabric between the cups, laid flat against the breastbone in front. The cups were filled out but not spilling over. The back band was parallel to the floor, not riding up. Upon raising my arms nothing budged. Check, check, and check.

I managed about 10 minutes in it before wanting to gasp. I felt anxious. I imagined being squeezed by an anaconda wrapped around my ribcage. I saw that on TV once, not the bra, just the anaconda. Marlon Perkins wrestled an anaconda on Mutual of Omaha's Wild Kingdom right in our living room. I believe he won because that is how my brother and I acted it out for years to come. Standing in the bathroom curiosity still called to me and I decided to wrestle into the other bra. The "32-inch" model was an acute insult to my lungs. It also "fit" right. No gaps, no bulges. But, I had to exhale most of the time. Here is the biggest point. When I actually measured the length of the bra band it was 26 inches! The 34-inch model was 28 inches. Of course it did not fit my ribs, lungs, and heart even if it "fit" by mannequin standards. I tried adding a bra extender or two, but it really needed nearly 3 of the 2-inch extenders to be a healthy circumference. Alas, they were returned.

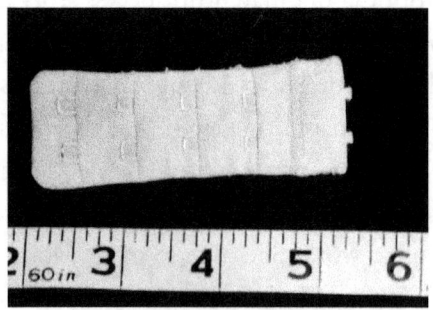

Figure 5.1: 2-inch Bra extender
An extender can add approximately 2 inches to a bra band. The recommended bra size needed 3 extenders to breathe comfortably!

There is a lack of consistency in the measuring and sizing system. I call it full of creativity, with a touch of fantasy. As clothing consumers we likely have 3 or more clothing size labels in our closets. What makes bra sizing so much more challenging is the intimacy of the bra, the challenge of being exposed, vulnerable, and measuring up to ever shifting ideals of worthiness. This section and the later chapter are focused on knowledge as power. To feel confident in your own uniqueness and choose to wear what fits you best physically and socially. That choice may or may not include a traditional bra.

Shortly, we will peruse the various bra measurements, sizing, and fitting I found online and in person with professional fitters.

Before we take measurements for a bra, let's consider measurements for our health. We'll learn about our breath and how it is measured in the western medical physiology and its importance to all healing traditions. In the coming chapters we will introduce the relationship of breath to mental balance, and fluid movement.

6

Measurements for Health

Years ago, in my frustration with bra bands, I decided to measure my ribcage at rest and then after exercise. I had several years of daily yoga and breathing practice at that time and I was more and more aware of the range of motion of my chest wall. Pre-exercise measurements were made in the morning at rest, before my morning routine. I made a second set of measurements after yoga and a vigorous walk.

I measured 3 times at the level of the bra band and then calculated the average for that position. Measurements were made with a full exhalation followed by a second set holding a full breath in. I took the big number and subtracted the little number to see how much my chest needed to expand for a full breath. I did it to prove to myself that a bra band can't physically change size like a healthy human and to tell anyone who would listen.

Upon first waking the difference between inhalation and exhalation was 2 ¾ inches. After yoga, pranayama (yogic breathing practice), and a brisk walk in nature my chest wall excursion was nearly 4 inches! A full breath out to a full breath in made a 12% change from my resting chest measurement. I ran for my bra drawer. I made measurements of the band at resting length and again stretched it as far as possible. No go. I exercised them a bit, stretching and pulling. Nothing. The underwire in one seemed to poke out more, so I pulled it out. The change in length of the bra bands ranged from 1 ¾ to 3 inches. But, there was a lot of recoil in the tissue, the fabric I mean. It really wanted to be at its resting length all day whereas a living ribcage enjoys a resting "neutral" at several different circumferences.

In her book, *Breath*, Belisa Vranich, PhD describes a breathing "grade" based on similar measurements. The initial goal she sets is a 10% change in circumference with full inhalation and exhalation. A shortcut to this calculation is to move the decimal one space to the left from your resting measurement.

Here is an example:

> If the resting circumference of the chest below the breast is 30 inches a 10% change between inhalation and exhalation would be 3 inches.
> 10% of 30 = 3 OR 30.0 move the decimal becomes 3.0
> Measuring the same place with the breath fully inhaled and breath fully exhaled may look like this:
> Full inhalation: 32 inches
> Full exhalation: 29 inches
> 32-29=3
> This chest wall's measurements would meet the goal of a 10% change.

A more formal medical measurement of respiratory function (how well you are breathing) is called a Pulmonary Function Test or PFT.

During medical school, I was running or biking daily and generally appeared fit and healthy. As second-year students we set up pulmonary function tests in the physiology lab to really see how these measurements were made. Then we tested ourselves. I recall my physiology professor, also a distance runner, beaming during the successful lab. He came to my table expecting to show off some great readings (to validate distance running and lung fitness, no doubt!) His face fell with disappointment. The numbers weren't stellar. I thought I would be asked to repeat the lab as my professor was sure there had been an error. Sharing a history of pneumonia including chemical pneumonia from first-year anatomy lab (preservatives are not for living lungs), I told him, "I'm doing the best with what I have." With a flash of insight and an approving nod, he moved on to the next table.

Ten years later I had a regular home yoga practice, albeit 15 minutes a day, and a walking, not running, routine. On a slow (due to snow) day at my second job I asked our nurse to run me through the spirometry test we used for physicals. Spirometry measures several of the parameters that a PFT does, but not quite as complete. New PFT and spirometry machines also print an "interpretation" including a calculated "lung age." Imagine my surprise to see "Lung-age: 21 years". I was 33. I knew my breathing had felt easier the last 2 years and I had experienced fewer coughs and colds. I surmised it had to do with my breathing practice in yoga poses and pranayama. I also became aware that when my breathing and temperament felt at its best, my bra band felt its worst. It was too snug and bothersome. The reverse became an indicator of stress for me as well. When my bra was not bothersome tight I realized I had tension in my life and breath.

Therefore when my bra band felt comfortable, I scheduled an osteopathic treatment for my ribs and diaphragm as they had "locked-up" and I was not breathing as fully. Right after a treatment, the bra band felt snug again. (Don't worry, I unhooked it) Hence, I was prompted to get the tape measure and make those pre and post-exercise measurements!

Measurements and design

We will delve into the world of multiple measurements and calculators momentarily. But, have you ever wondered why we measure bras like batteries, triple A to double D?

According to Laura Tempesta's TEDx talk, *You'll Never Look at a Bra the Same Way Again*, bra sizing came from Victorian shirt sizing of the 1800s. This morphed to standard "band and cup" sizing with band size in imperial inches. Cup size was given a letter, just like batteries,

AAA, AA, A, B, C, D, and DD/E, F, G, and so on. A common misconception is that a bigger cup letter means more cup volume. This is an easy assertion and understandable misconception. But, what we don't realize is band and cup sizes are linked. As band size decreases cup letter increases to keep the same volume. For instance, a 36 C cup volume is comparable to the cup volume to a 34D in that bra maker's specific style. The notion that bigger letters mean bigger breasts is so prevalent that we hear it spoken by women as well as men in our culture. "I'm a D cup" (often said with dismay by women while shopping for swimwear) or "Ooh, double D's" (spoken without dismay near the swimwear section) Whether it is misconception fueling designers or designers catering to public misconception, it is my opinion that the misunderstanding of the linked band and cup measurements has led to the multitude of "correct" ways to measure for a bra found today on the internet.

The most widely accepted method by fitters and designers alike employs a "5-inch" calculation. A trained bra fitter in a specialty or department store will measure the circumference above the breasts up under the armpit and around the fullest part of the bust. These measurements are usually taken standing while wearing a bra or even over clothes. The band size is determined by adding 5 inches to the underarm measurement. Cup size is determined by subtracting the calculated band size from the bust measurement and then referring to a table to find the correlating cup letter. A 1-inch difference is an "A" cup, a 2-inch difference equals a "B" cup, and a 3-inch difference correlates to a "C" cup. After measuring and calculating, an experienced, thoughtful retailer will bring you a variety of options in your size range including a few "equivalent sizes" such as 36C and 34D in the same style. None of these options will actually measure 36 or 34 inches in band length but will measure 4-8 inches shorter even in the same brand, resulting in a garment about 28 inches in band circumference.

There are a few inherent errors to this method. To use the "5-inch" value as a mathematical constant in an equation means it must hold true for any height or weight woman. If this is true for women 4"10" to 6'2" then it must continue to be true when applied to the extremes.

To visualize this imagine a Barbie doll at 12-inch height and Ella Ewing, the tallest woman on record, at 8 feet 4 ½ inches. Barbie's calculation of adding 5 inches is just silly, the tape falls to the floor with our beliefs. Only allowing 5 inches to Ella's measurements places her heart and lungs in a bind. Therefore, the 5-inch constant isn't a true constant. So, why is it used? The 5-inch measurement was designed to fit a specific mold, a ratio of desired proportion at that time in history, regardless of height or frame. Now that we know more about the origin and intention of measuring systems, we can free up to develop something that actually functions well for an individual.

In my research for a healthier bra, I encountered a TED talk by the owner of Vibrant Bra, Michael Drescher. His presentation on bras, health, and culture is worth a look. I contacted the small company and was introduced to their delightful designer, Heidi Lehman. Heidi is a lingerie designer from Germany who came to find herself in Milwaukee with a few stops along the way. She hosts virtual fittings for bras and underclothes she creates. I signed up online with a friend and prepared my notepad. Such a wealth of information she shared. I learned how she grades the sizes of bands and cups in her two styles of bras and that not all companies use exactly the same grading or "sister sizing". She also explained how different colors of fabric affect the fit of the bra. Darker dyes make fabric less stretchy making them fit tighter. With decades of experience in the lingerie industry, Heidi commented on the lag in design compared to the changing shape of women's bodies, fuller and more muscular in particular. She recognizes the difference in a more circular chest wall versus square or rectangular as well as the overall variation in size. We did a virtual fitting taking measurements that aligned with her designs and noting the whole shape of the torso. I will share how to take those measurements shortly. The experience felt pleasingly couture! In the end, we must remember that bras are already made. Although we made custom measurements I did not order a custom brassiere. Measuring is only to find a starting point to see which one you may fit in. Not, which one is made to fit you. The take-home point here is to not be concerned with numbers and letters. Be concerned with whether the bra meets your goals and standards. This one met my standards for clean, non-toxic materials (all OEKO-Tex Standard-100 certified), wire free, and aesthetically pleasing. But, it did not meet my goal of easy breath and ribcage movement. If the bra were a pair of shoes I would put them on the special occasion shelf, pretty and well-crafted. I would try to wear them more often but keep finding them under the dinner table next to my toes.

The Measurements

I suspect you are going to head to the internet and be faced with a multitude of well-meaning bra-fitting videos. You are in a much better place now to determine "fact" from "farce." The following is a sampling of such findings with the light of insight shining into them. The best measurements would be without numbers. An unmarked string to compare your dimensions to the article of clothing you are considering wearing is my best recommendation.

Below are two different systems for measuring I've tried. I prefer these two systems as they both emphasize measuring on bare skin, not over clothing or another bra. Heidi's method has the more unique "over the hill" measurement which can help match up breast volume to a specific cup. A friend clued me in to another approach. The measurements recommended by ABraThatFits.org utilize three positions recognizing that there is a living, breathing *person* behind the breasts. I would modify the loose, snug and tight measurements to correspond to full inhalation, neutral breath and exhalation.

Heidi's method of measure

1. Ribcage below breasts to determine band size
2. Under the arms and above breasts +5" (to confirm the band size)
3. Breast tissue measurement from the side of the breast under the arm to the center of chest or where breast tissue ends. An "over the hill" measurement for cup size related to band size.

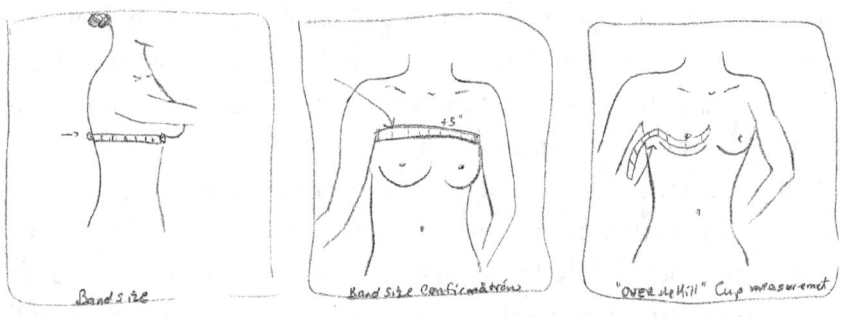

Figure 6.1: Designer's Measurement System
Measurements from left to right are Band Size, Band Size Confirmation, and Over the Hill Cup Measurement.

ABraThatFits.org

1. Make 3 measurements at the bust line: standing, bending forward at the waist. and lying face up
2. Measure over bare skin at the chest below breasts: loose, snug, and tight.
3. A size is calculated in US or UK size by entering the measurements into their online calculator.

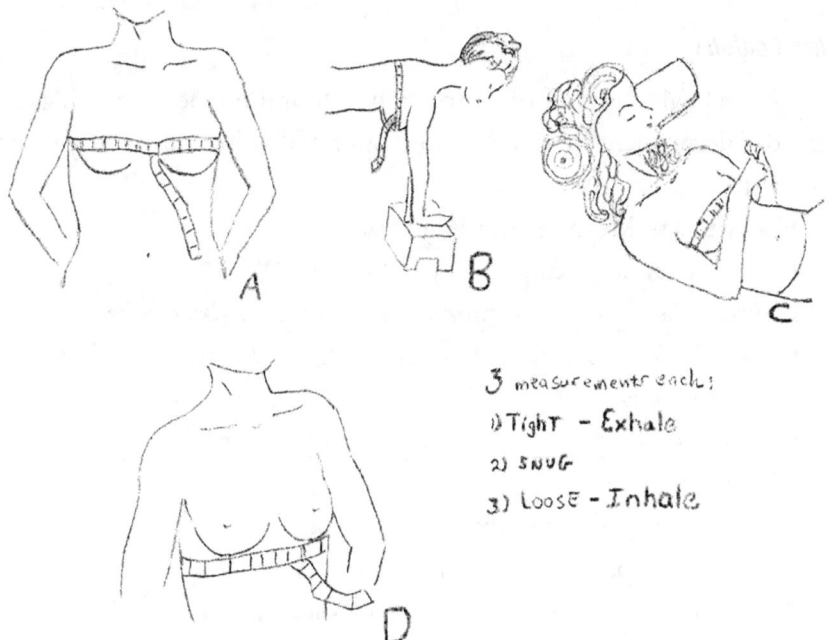

Figure 6.2: ABraThatFits.org Suggested Measurements
Tight, loose, and snug measurements are taken in each of the four positions shown: standing bustline, leaning forward, supine, and standing chest below breast.

My internet foray to clarify the 5-inch constant for determining bra band size was quite a shock. Between department stores, lingerie stores, and YouTube® home videos on bra-fitting there was no pattern for "how-to measure" and the resulting "size recommendations." A few days later I resolved to sort it out with a friend.

Using measurements described in the more inclusive ABraThatFits.org to enter into other online calculators we recorded the results. Recommended sizes ranged from 36 AA to 32EE! A rainbow of letters filled in between 34 C, 34 D, and 32 E. And, to give us a giggle one site concluded in bright red letters "We're having trouble finding your size. Try again or visit your nearest store."

Avoid pitfalls

The following is a set of instructions I found online from a highly-regarded department store. I will point out pitfalls especially as they relate to health:

How (not) to Measure Your Band Size
• Put on your best-fitting, non-padded bra.

If there were a great fitting, unpadded bra in the dresser these instructions may not be necessary. The real concern for this recommendation is taking measurements over a bra. I recommend measurements over the skin.

• Wrap a measuring tape snugly around your rib cage, just beneath your bust line.

Snug? My oxygen meters are going off already.

• Adjust the tape so that it's parallel to the floor. *Okay*
• Exhale deeply—you want the smallest measurement possible.

Uh-oh! This looks like measuring for a corset. Now is the time to think, do you want to only exhale while wearing it?

• Round to the nearest whole number and refer to the size chart. *Darn, after all that it's only an estimate.*

And, how (not) to measure your **cup** size:
"Refer to the bra you are wearing for the cup size."

Does it "fit"?

An internet exploration of "Does your bra fit correctly?" reveals a little more consistency than the measuring-to-be-fitted process. But, does it *really* fit? Well, that all comes down to the checklist now, doesn't it? In Chapter 5 I described my experience with nearly professional measurements, ordering, and a video tutorial checklist. I say "nearly professional" due to my growing up experience with professional fitters in department stores, the garments and the associated tutorial were of high quality and I dare to say any professional fitter would have been very pleased with the result. But, this is a book about health and empowering knowledge. My dream-bra checklist was not met with the garment despite the high quality, and here is why, there is a different "checklist" for health.

Multiple sites and videos reviewed how to determine fit and I found these parameters were more consistent than the how-to-measure-for-fit sites. But I do not agree with the physics when used on human bodies versus a mannequin's noncompressible trunk.

Most videos reference that 80% of "support" comes from the band. Others cite "90%"? (Studies prove that 87% of statistical percentages are made up on the spot.) The point was that the bra band was recommended to be *tight* around the ribcage in order to have a fixed point from which to leverage and lift (support) breasts off the front. But, the fixed point is your soft innards, heart and lungs. Worried about back fat bulging? Amazingly enough you can see before and after images of wearing a *tighter* band to prevent the bra from sliding up in back producing a bulge. This works on mannequins for two reasons. First, the solid form does not give in to pressure nor need to breathe. Second, the majority of mannequins have an "hourglass" figure, the ribcage funnels down to the smallest point at the waist. Not all women are this shape and some shapes are the inverse with a larger waist than bust.

Wearing a bra or any strap pressed into tissue acts like a removable scar. In the next chapter, I will discuss scars and their influence on the health of our body's systems. To trained hands the sensation of scar tissue feels like chronic restriction in the energy and fluid fields of the body. Scars can also decrease range of motion in joints and restrict organ function.

You are creating your own priorities now and will be forming your own personalized "checklists" to produce the results you want.

Special Concerns

Pre-teens and teens

My thoughts for pre-teens and teens are simple. Recognize that this is a time to fit in with your peers. Choose your peers carefully, and your bras, too. To bra or not to bra should fit you as an individual. Be your own trend-setter!

I will address 3 special points for adolescence in this section:

- Hormone production tied to environmental toxins
- EMFs as a toxin and how to reduce the load
- Growth stimulated by hormone production and the restrictive effects of "training bras on overall growth"

Pre-puberty through adolescence marks a time of rapid production of some particular hormones; estrogen, progesterone, DHEA, and testosterone. These hormones are built from special fats in our body and from fats we eat. The better the dietary balance of "good" fats and low toxins the more efficient the hormone production pathway can be and the transition from young girl to grown woman complete with curves. Curves are smoothed out by fat which plays a role in energy storage but is also a reservoir for toxins. This book is about breast curves. Breasts are formed of breast tissue and filled out with fat to form the curves. Developing breast tissue with its companion fat tissue is more susceptible to toxins as the tissues are in a growing phase.

This is a particularly good time in life to be aware of toxins in clothing lying next to skin. Toxins range from chemicals added on after production such as insect repellent for moths during shipping to chemicals that are inherent in the materials, pesticides and herbicides sprayed on cotton fields, and out-gassing of synthetic materials such as polyurethane foam used to mold cups of bras. Chemicals are absorbed through skin and milk duct openings of the nipple. Chemical exposure combined with squeezed lungs and lymph drainage creates a challenge to cells' detoxification at any age!

Another source of toxins is in the rapidly increasing sea of electromagnetic radiation through electromagnetic fields or EMFs. There are three main classes of EMFs based on the wavelength of the energy: electrical, magnetic, and radiofrequency. Metal attracts electrical fields, that's how lightning rods work in a storm. Metal also acts like an antenna and amplifies electrical fields. But, surprising new research shows radiofrequency, a much higher frequency, to affect tissues around metal as well. Specifically, research has shown increased leakage around metal dental fillings between the filling and tooth structure with cell phone use next to the head. Cell phones themselves have both an antenna and transmitter with the signal strength of a cell tower. Really, go figure, it has to get the signal all the way back to the tower. EMF education is very important so we can choose to use it wisely. Bottom line for teens and the rest of us, keep the cell phone off the body. Reduce the amount of signal emitted by closing apps when not in use, and turning off Bluetooth, wifi, or cell when not in use. Use airplane mode to stop radiofrequencies when you don't have or need reception. And, it now seems obvious; do not carry a cell phone in your bra.

Breasts grow during adolescence but so does everything! Consider bones, muscles, brain, heart, and lungs to set the stage. Starting with bones and bras, the ribs and spine are making their final growth spurt to adult length. They are extra flexible and can easily be compressed at the expense of the heart and lungs beneath them. This is such an important time to be sure our girls are able to grow strong through their chest wall for a healthy heart and lungs. Take extra care choosing an athletic bra as well. Developing breast tissue can be extra tender, even painful with exercise movements. This is a time to look for wider coverage in a sports bra to wear during high-impact activities and to remove or loosen it when you are not.

In the book *The Rules* (for dating) co-authors Ellen Fein and Sherry

Schneider introduce the concept of being a "CUAO," a Creature Unlike Any Other. Funny ladies. The authors recommend you show up as *your* best self, a true Creature Unlike Any Other. They recognize that people, especially men, love knowing they have the "special one." I agree! Playing on your uniqueness as your strength is a double blessing. And although pre-teen and teen years are a natural time for fitting in, it's never too early to impress this concept of strength in uniqueness.

"You will never be better than ME, you can only be the best YOU! And vice-versa" to quote a colleague, Andrew Lovy, D.O.

Pregnancy and Breastfeeding

Pregnancy is a time of growth and more growth. Baby is growing, occupying more and more space. First the pelvis, then the abdomen, and finally the thoracic space itself is partially occupied with this new creation. Meanwhile, Mom's own tissues are developing. Uterine muscle multiplies, the lining grows, and breasts increase in size with glandular development. Between baby-occupied territory and her own tissue acquisitions, the maternal-fetal unit changes shape and size daily for almost 2 years! Once again I've seen a few impressive bras, but this calls for more.

Consider your goals during this time. The rapid breast growth and fluid retention of pregnancy can result in painful breasts and you may want to wear a bra or modified "breast brace". I recommend non-toxic fabrics, and balancing the amount of immobilization needed for comfort with the most amount of ease in motion for ribs and diaphragm. An inexpensive pair of bra extenders can save the day as circumference changes and allow a bra to be worn further into pregnancy if desired.

Breastfeeding brings its own set of goals. Non-toxic components next to skin and baby are a priority as is the ability for the bra or undershirt to accommodate changes in breast size throughout the day. Hard construction bras such as those with underwires or side stays are a potential cause of painful clogged milk ducts. Cups that are too small and press into the top of the breast tissue can obstruct milk ducts as well. Clogged ducts can lead to an infection called mastitis that is best avoided.

Lastly, be sure bra cups and nursing pads are thoroughly dry after washing. The thick layers of organic cotton or wool flannel can take some time to dry. Lay them in sunlight for a bit to deter fungal growth. Extra moisture in breast pads can lead to a painful fungal overgrowth like candida thrush on Mom's nipple and baby's tongue.

Breast tissue swelling from many causes have seen rapid relief with osteopathic treatment of drainage pathways. The breast care section of this book will give you self-care tools based on osteopathic principles you can use at home.

II

Under it all

7

Anatomy: A New Perspective

"You begin with anatomy, and you end with anatomy, a knowledge of anatomy is all you want or need."
Andrew Taylor Still, M.D., D.O., Philosophy of Osteopathy

Have you wondered what other body parts could be affected by placing a tight band around the chest? In Section II you have the opportunity to skim the surface or dive into anatomical form and function.

Chapter 7 reveals layers like old-fashioned transparencies, lifting off each superficial layer to see what's underneath. Chapter 8 elaborates on the details of anatomy interlacing a fresh perspective on physiology with Eastern and Western views and personal accounts.

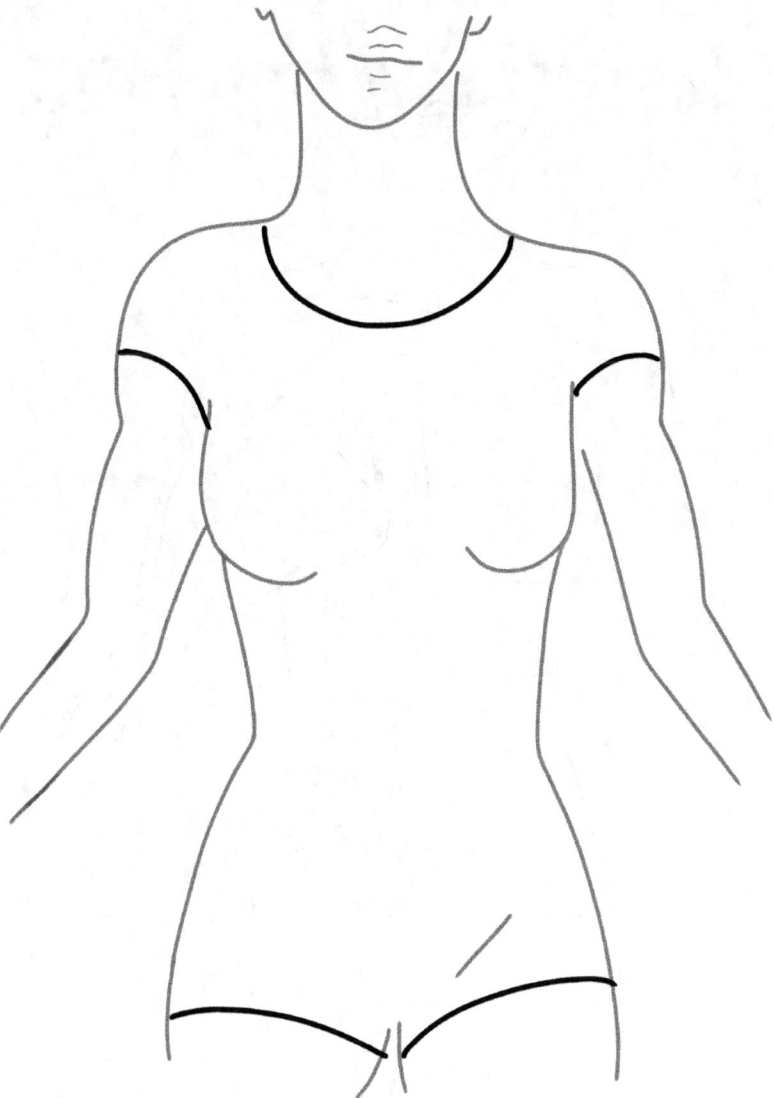

Figure 7.1: Female Form

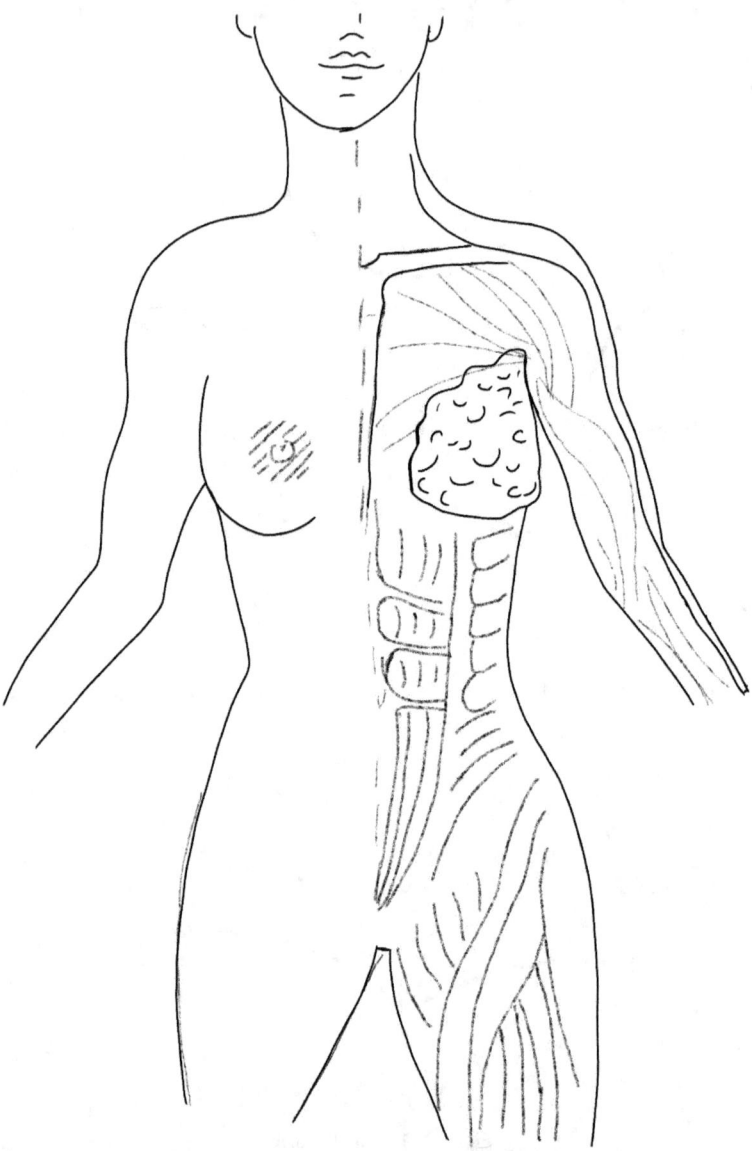

Figure 7.2: Skin and Muscle Layers
Skin, areola and nipple are seen on the model's right side. The skin on the left side has been lifted away to show the breast gland interspersed with fat and the musculature under the fascia.

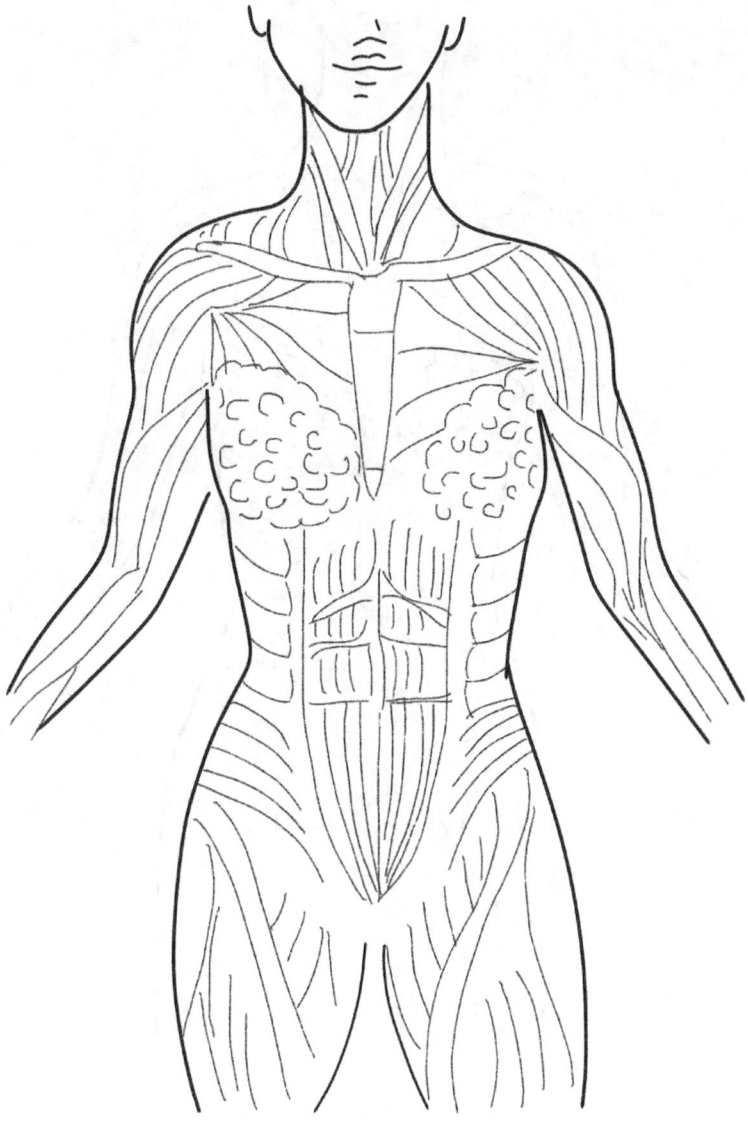

Figure 7.3: Muscular System
Both sides of the skin and superficial fascia have been removed to show the network of muscles and position of breast glands.

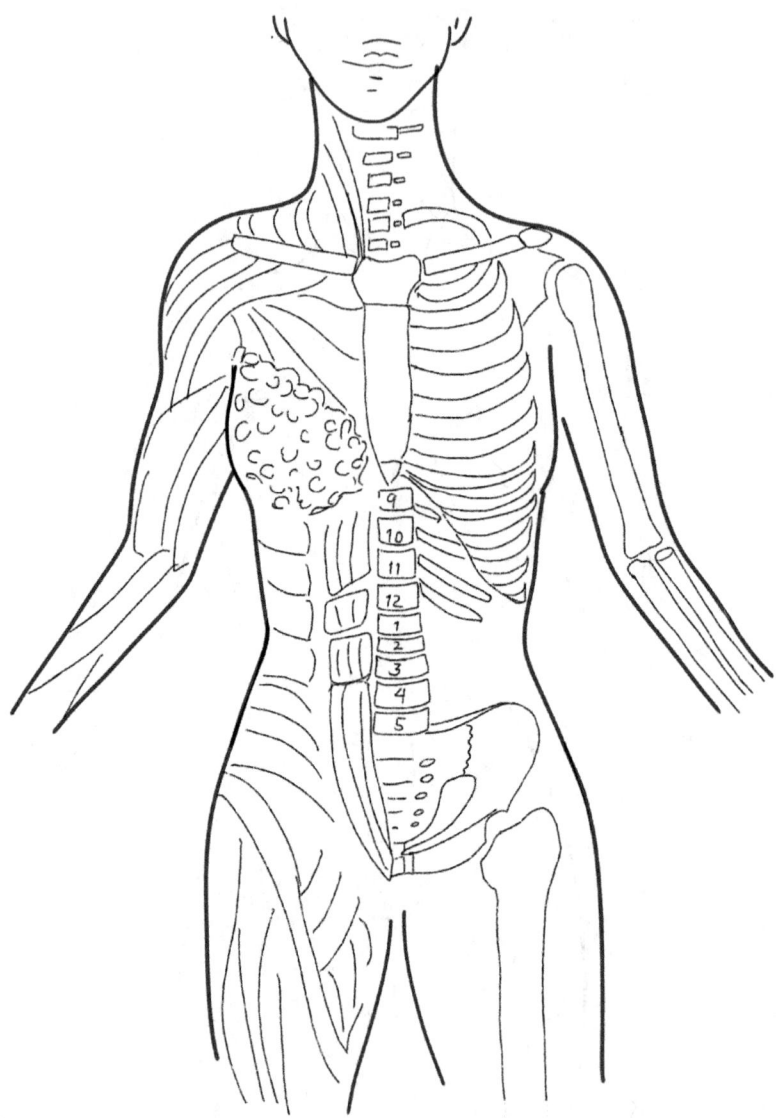

Figure 7.4: Muscle and Bone
Here the muscular layer has been removed down to the bone on the model's left side and the muscular layer on the model's right side remains. Note the collarbones (clavicles), breastbone (sternum), ribs, thoracic and lumbar spine with numbers, sacrum, pelvis and hip joint.

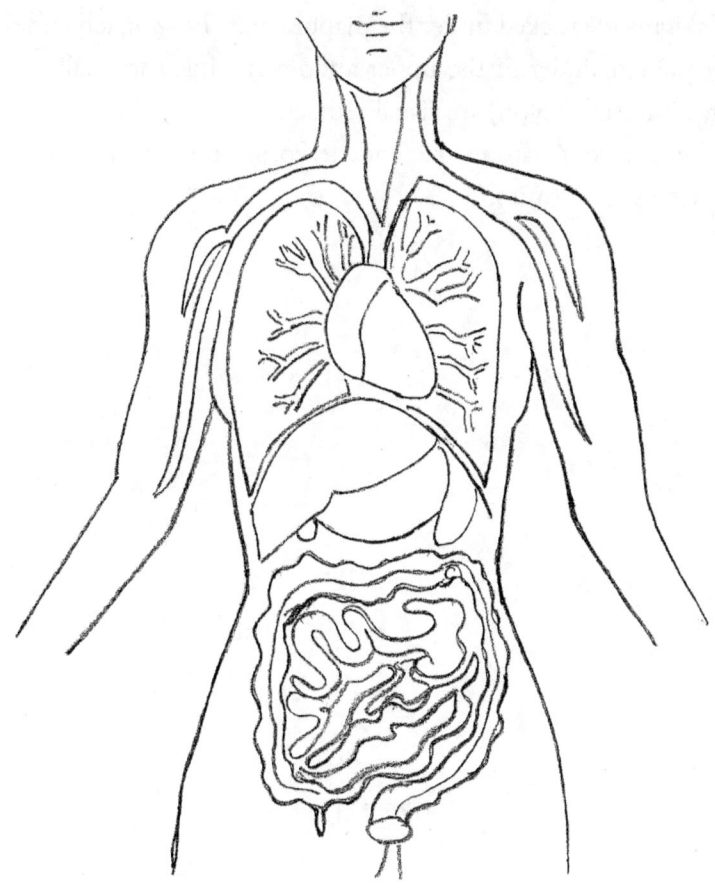

Figure 7.5: Internal Organs
The heart, lungs, liver, stomach, spleen, small intestine, and colon are revealed.

Shazam! All the way down to the internal organs. Under the bony ribcage we see the heart in the center of the chest spiraling to a point angled to the model's left. Lungs and bronchi branch out from center to outer chest. The chest cavity is separated from the abdominal and pelvic organs by the thoraco-abdominal diaphragm. It is usually referred to as "the diaphragm" but, there are more than one as you will find in Chapter 8.

In the abdomen and pelvis you see the large domed liver on the model's right side tucked under the diaphragm. The stomach and spleen occupy the remainder of the upper abdomen while the small intestine and large intestine (colon) are visualized below.

Follow me to Anatomy Expanded: Form and Function for more depth, details, and stories.

8

Anatomy Expanded: Form and Function

Electrical and energy systems

Just when you thought the inside and the outside were plenty to study, we are introduced to "outside" the outside. The what? It's the space around yourself you call "my space". "Hey, you're in my space" space. It is also where we find the bio-electrical field associated with the body's own electrical system. Subtle energy, such as aura/wei chi and meridians are described here and this energy also perfuses the inside of anatomy. Since the energy aspect of anatomy is present in all organs, cells, and the fluid they are bathed in we will start here!

Electric

Lying face-up and relaxed on my treatment table was a young woman in her 20s. She was receiving an osteopathic cranial treatment. Osteopathy in the cranial field is a form of osteopathic treatment for the whole body that can be very potent but feel very subtle. During the treatment, while standing at the foot of the table, I was surprised to perceive a stream of

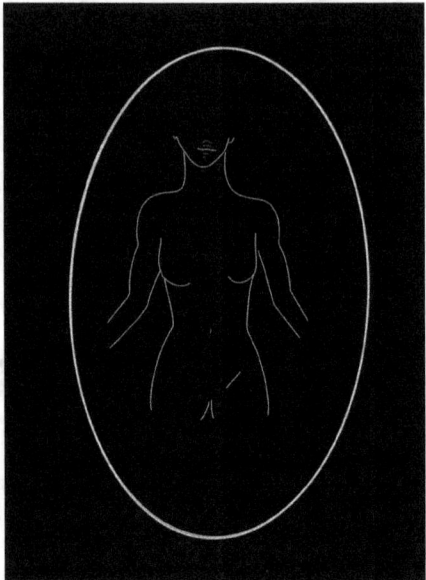

Figure 8.1: Bio-energetic Field
The bio-energetic field is represented by a 3-D, egg-shaped energetic field surrounding the body.

light that flowed from the big toe of her right foot up to her chest. It was about 3mm wide and the luminous color of liquid sunlight. Upon reaching her bra band the light stream fragmented and scattered across her breast. The fragments of light dissipated never re-forming into a stream. Hmm, I thought, a mystery to solve.

I had just started my studies of TCM (Traditional Chinese Medicine) and meridians and I was beginning to memorize meridians by images in textbooks. What I saw looked so much like the liver meridian but it was not "textbook." Instead, I was reminded of a CT scan of the head when there are metal dental fillings in the teeth. The result is a scattering of light in the images called "artifact." The shards of brilliant white artifact obliterate parts of the image. Artifact distorts the information and limits interpretation by a radiologist.

Was there metal in or on the patient scattering the stream of light energy?

"Are you wearing an underwire bra?" I inquired.

"Yes, all of my bras are underwire," she confirmed.

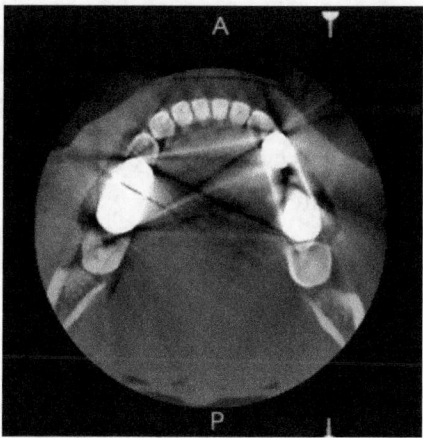

Figure 8.2: Dental CT with Scatter Refraction from Crowns

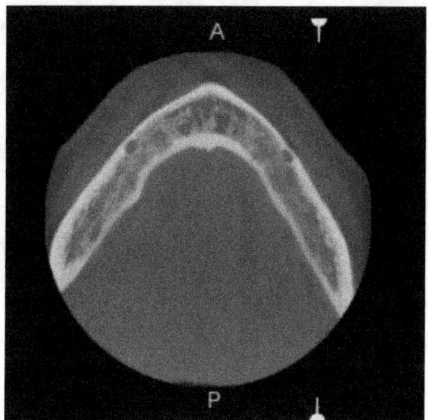

Figure 8.3: Dental CT of Mandible without Refraction.

Oh dear, I thought. I really can't ignore this! Had metal hardware fractured information in the light? Was the body able to interpret the scattered information correctly? If the light I saw was a page of instructions, it was as though the paper had been torn up and tossed about.

Years later I would study electrical fields of both our bodies and our environment to discover the antennae effect of metal on our bodies while in an electrical field. Underwire bras definitely count as antennae. Even wireless bras can have metal in clasps, shoulder straps and decorations. Consulting with a building biologist I learned that we unintentionally are exposed to electrical fields every day in our own homes and buildings. I also learned how to mitigate it.

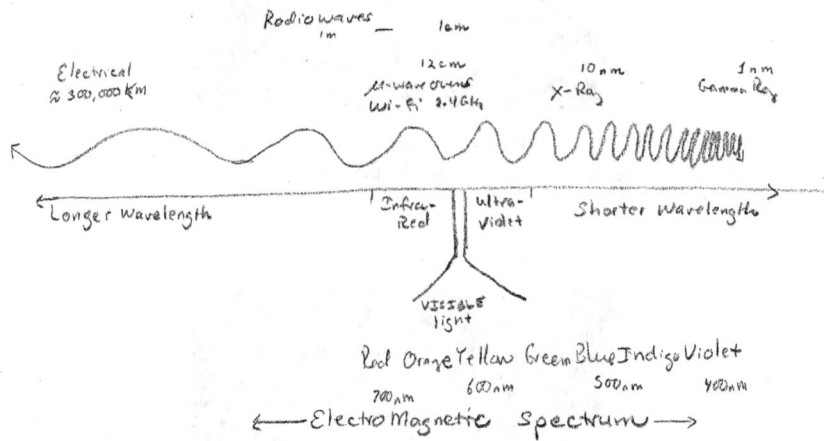

Figure 8.4: Electromagnetic Spectrum
The electromagnetic spectrum displays wavelengths from long to short. An electrical field waveform would stretch from the east to west coast of the U.S. Visible light is a tiny slice in the middle and very short waveforms include x-ray and gamma rays used in the medical field.

Electrical fields are produced by electrical wiring in our homes, offices, and outdoors under electric lines. In household wiring, the field extends about 6 feet. This includes wiring in the walls, ceiling, and floor. Any metal within this 6-foot field acts like a lightning rod attracting and expanding the electrical field. The electrical energy frequency range is described as extremely low frequency or ELF with a wavelength cycling at 50 to 60 Hertz. This cycle is a back-and-forth oscillation that occurs 50-60 times per second. Iron-rich red blood cells are particularly vulnerable to electrical fields. As the oscillating field pulls on the iron it wiggles the blood cells 60 times per second. (60Hz for electricity in the U.S. and 50Hz for Europe.) Nerve tissue and the conductive system of the heart are also susceptible to electrical fields due to their conductive nature.

"EMF" and "EMFs" are the abbreviations for both electromagnetic fields and electromagnetic frequencies. Although not analogous, they are often used interchangeably.

Native EMFs describe electromagnetic frequencies and fields that occur in nature. Our bodies are electric and produce a native electromagnetic field. Sunlight, also a native source of EMF, carries the full spectrum of visible light as well as infrared and ultraviolet rays. A light bulb however emits only part of the spectrum (it ain't natural). Our human bodies are electric, naturally native to us. Anywhere on or off the body an electrical charge can be measured. The heart's electrical conduction can be seen in an EKG or electrocardiogram. Think of a movie where the hospital scene shows a monitor with the heartbeat tracing. A rhythmic sequence of the heart's electric field is seen as a line going along straight up, down, and bump. A series of different "views" of the heart's electrical flow make up an EKG. *Here is the interesting part, the tracing changes when the body's electrical flow is presented with scar tissue.* Electricity cannot pass through it so it finds the shortest path around the scar. Why the importance of scar tissue? 'Cause bras and bands act like scar tissue. The electrical energy and subtle energy have to find a way around it. Like the shattered light I saw over the breast of the young woman wearing an underwire bra.

Electrical and subtle energy travels in the path of least resistance. Scars, metal, and compression create distortion to flow. Bra metals and mechanical pressure behave like scar tissue and can even cause scarring! Shoulder strap grooves, for instance, are formed by long-term pressure on skin and soft tissue over shoulder bones. Pressure causes tissue necrosis (death of cells). In my hospital days, I recall examining patients' backsides daily to check for pressure ulcers also known as bedsores where the body was pressed into the mattress too long.

You just completed a crash course in physics! Let's move on to the softer side of science, subtle energy. I suppose it is called "subtle" since it seems elusive and difficult to measure or see. Some see and know it easily, some want to quantify it to be seen and others deny its existence. One wonders what makes the presence of subtle energy any different than the presence of electricity before we had tools and technology to measure it. Before we harnessed electricity, wiring our homes, cities, and even our cars, it was present. Static charge zapping the kiss under mistletoe, lightning splitting the night sky are displays of electricity in nature. Subtle energy was there, too.

Thoughts and feelings are forms of subtle energy with effects far from unnoticeable. A pleasant visualization or thought of an image can cascade to a reduced heart rate, dilated blood vessels, and lowered blood pressure. And we have all witnessed the glow of someone in love.

Traditional Chinese Medicine reflects what we learn in the model: blood flow follows energy flow or qi to an area and energy is led there by thought or attention. I really appreciate this model as it adds an additional layer to western physiology without competing. TCM recognizes the electrical system as well. We are not as accustomed to seeing graphs of meridian energy flow. These frequencies of the body's energy are referred to as subtle energy as well. The meridians are all interconnected forming a highway that changes names as it passes through different "cities" or organs. For example, we have a Heart organ and a Heart meridian, a Small Intestine organ, and a Small Intestine meridian. It is one long meridian changing names as it flows into the next section of service. A road may change names as it crosses into a different section of town. It's the same road passing new geography. A meridian and its associated organ share some geographic proximity and support one another.

What was that luminous light on the patient? Was it subtle energy I perceived behaving in a predictable way following the laws of physics in electricity? "Unknown unknowns." Recognizing that unknowns exist even if we don't know about them is the first step to discovery. For example, if I had not seen an image or two of meridians in a book and then the streak of light during a patient encounter, I may not have "seen the light." I might have disregarded it as the lighting in the room, or just not acknowledged it at all. How many unknown unknowns do we miss when we think we know what we are looking for? Chris Voss calls these

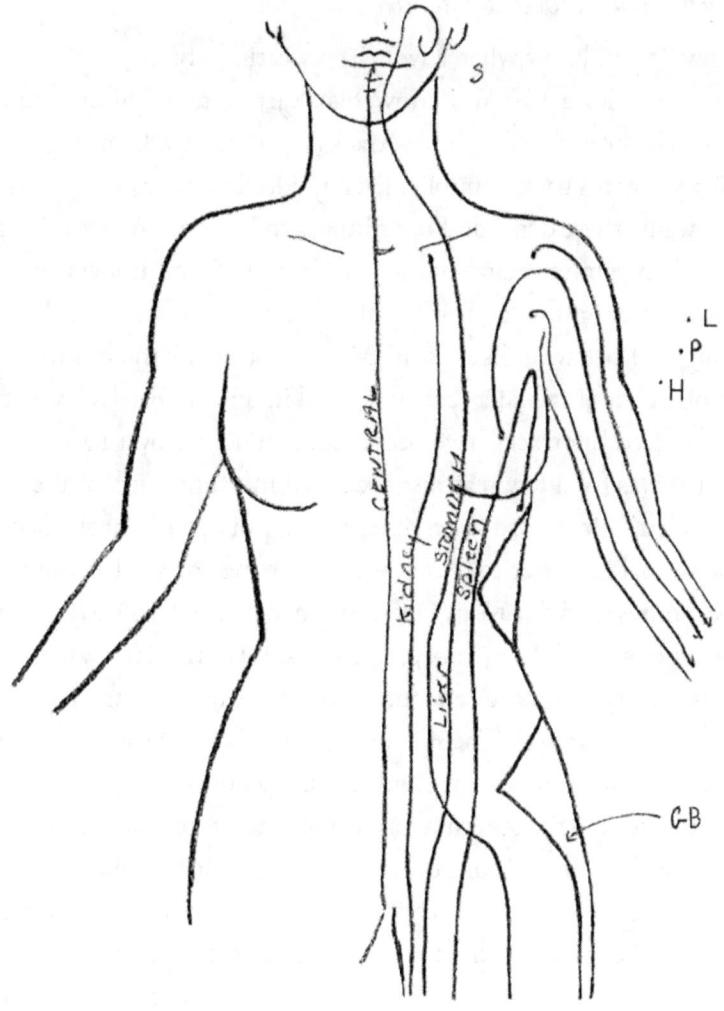

Figure 8.5: Twelve Main Meridians
The meridians are mirrored on both sides of the body; only one side is shown in this image. Labeled meridians are Central, Kidney, Stomach, Liver, Spleen, Gallbladder (GB), Heart (H), Pericardium (P), and Lung (L).

unknown unknowns "Black Swans" in his book Never Split the Difference, a realistic and holistic manual on communication and negotiation. Read on to see how our energy system interacts with and supports all of our tissues through the extracellular matrix.

Skin, scars, and extracellular matrix

How do you know when a woman is wearing a bra?

It's the "bra tracks." You know, like "carpet tracks" after vacuuming the rug. Subconsciously, these "tracks" are the mark of a good bra-wearing woman's back in public. Even if, ideally, every bra-fitter and bra-wearer wants these dents and back bulges to be gone! We even have bras marketed to minimize appearance of "back fat" and underarm bulges. Whether curvy, muscular, thick or thin the marks are there, visible under clothing and behaving like a scar. Movement causes the bra to tug and catch on fabric just like a scar tugs on skin and deeper layers of tissue. I have noticed bra tracks have become much deeper over past decades. I suspect this is for a few reasons: Increased measurements of the average American; a shift toward faster, cheaper shopping without the benefit of a professional bra-fitter to check fit; and progression of the compression bra becoming everyday wear. Decades ago, having an exposed bra or visible bra lines was a fashion faux pas. Let's aspire to that standard again!

Our skin is the first to encounter our clothing and its pressure, texture, chemicals, or dyes. The skin has multiple layers. From the outside in they are the epidermis, dermis, and subcutaneous tissues.

Skin structures the outermost aspect of the extracellular matrix (ECM). Interstitial fluid (fluid not contained in cells) floats amidst the fascial structure and the electrical energy flows through the collagen fibers.

Flattened dead skin cells form the epidermis that protects us from the environment and changes in temperature and moisture. The epidermis forms a protective coating over the deeper layer of dermis.

Dermis provides structure and strength to the skin and contains two layers, a loosely knit outer layer and denser under layer. It contains capillaries (tiny end vessels) and nerve fibers to supply the skin. Dermis also contains special cells called fibroblasts that help to knit-up wounds and form scars.

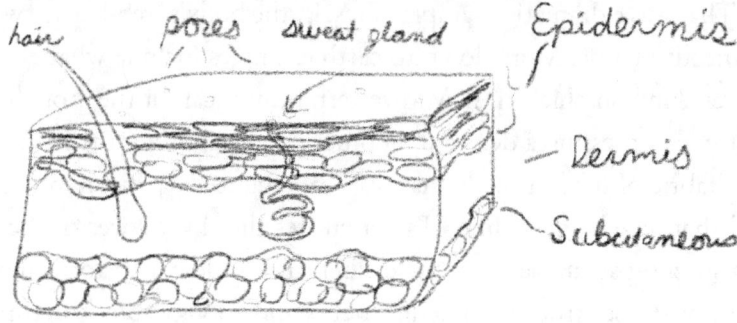

Figure 8.6: Cross-section of Skin
Layers of skin from superficial to deep are epidermis, dermis and subcutaneous tissue. Hair follicles and sweat glands penetrate the epidermis and dermis. The subcutaneous tissue is filled out with fat cell padding.

The subcutaneous tissue provides padding and fullness to the skin. Plump fat cells reside here. Constant pressure such as shoulder straps digging in causes tissue necrosis, in other words, death of the cells. This cell death results in tissue atrophy and tell-tale shoulder grooves as the tissue scars down. Plastic surgeons describe a procedure to fill in the shoulder grooves from bra straps by injecting fat cells into the divots. I would also recommend avoiding applying an offending strap again! Electrical and subtle energy travels in the path of least resistance. Scars create distortion to flow. Bra metals, pressure, and compression behave like scar tissue and can even cause scarring!

Fascia, scars, and the ECM

If all the cells of a person melted away you would still recognize a person. Eww, but true. That was one of my introductions to the intricacy of fascia over three decades ago. Since that time I have viewed amazing and unsettling research videos of the human heart being stripped of its cells, yes, muscle and nerve, everything, and the fascial template of the heart left behind. This "ghost heart" was then seeded with new cells.

That was a dramatic example of fascia, the body's web-like network of connective tissue. More down to earth examples include what chefs call "silver skin" on chicken. A Midwestern hunter calls it the "tough stuff" that makes dressing a deer out so much work. Your yoga teacher calls it the "fabric of life." (I made that up, I've taught yoga, but never actually said that, maybe next time.) Fascia creates the shiny cover of the meat. It also encapsulates each muscle fiber and coalesces to form tendons. It forms dense structures like ligaments and spongy soft structures like skin, breasts, and lungs. Fascia wraps and infuses each organ as we saw in the ghost heart. It provides tensegrity to our physical form. It is the structure that forms the extracellular matrix to support our interstitial fluid. You've probably heard humans are mostly water. It's true. But we are not a water balloon. We have intricate baffles formed of fascia. And, it is electrically conductive, almost sci-fi! A touch to any area of fascia lights up a radiating impulse through the body on the fascial highway. Whole books are written regarding approaches to the fascia in healing modalities including osteopathy, acupuncture, and yoga.

To get a sense of your own fascia, try this:

Step 1. Assess your shoulder motion. Raise your arms over your head first to the front and then to the side. Try to scratch your upper back with one hand and then the other. Notice how far you can reach in each position and how easy or tight the motion is to you.

Step 2. Massage the palm of one hand. Spend a relaxing moment to do it. Massage the center, the heel of the hand, and then down each finger. Stretch the hand open and closed.

Step 3. Re-check the range of motion in the arm with the freshly massaged hand. Compare to the other side.

Step 4. Repeat the massage for the other hand.

Step 5. Re-assess both sides. Repeat Step 1 to assess both sides after both hands are massaged. Did the first side have more change after both palms were addressed?

That sequence is inspired by yoga teacher Lilias Folan and I have used a version of it for flexibility training in my patients, and athletes for decades. It is based on the principle that the palms of the hands and soles of the feet are a fascial "bank" or storage. Accessing the bank allows the fascial fabric to lengthen and reach all the way up the arm and chest with ease. A similar sequence can be done for the soles of the feet resulting in greater ease of motion through the legs and lower back.

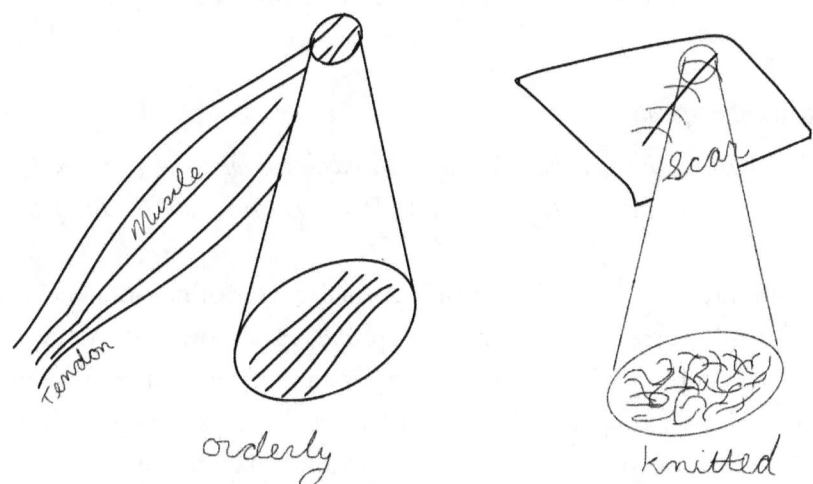

Figure 8.7: Collagen Fibers in Tendon and Scar Tissue
Both tendon and scar tissue are formed of collagen fibers. The parallel fibers of tendons and ligaments allow stretching and electrical flow. The densely knitted orientation of scar tissue interferes with electrical flow and restricts movement.

Like fascia, scar tissue is formed of collagen fibers as well. In this case the irregular fibers create a dense mass that does not conduct electricity well and interrupts the electrical system. It also tugs on the lattice work of the extracellular matrix affecting the movement of interstitial fluid, therefore the lymphatic system. Tension caused by scars can press over lymphatic channels affecting the flow of lymph in the vessels. Although scars are visible on the surface, deeper scar tissue forms as well in response to injury. For example, scar tissue forms in the heart after injury from a myocardial infarction, or heart attack. Adhesions are a type of scar tissue that may form in the abdomen from infection or after abdominal surgery. This is tough binding tissue. A classmate once revealed she had abdominal adhesions released and her height measured 3 inches taller afterward!

Breast tissue can scar, too. Multiple causes include injury such as striking the steering wheel or seat belt in an abrupt stop, infection known as mastitis, and surgical procedures of all types. Scars can inhibit energy and lymph flow. In Chapter 13, Breast-health and Self-care, tips are offered to optimize your body's and breasts' self-healing mechanisms.

Lymphatic system

"Thus we strike at the source of life and death when we go to the lymphatics."   Andrew Taylor Still, M.D., D.O., *Philosophy of Osteopathy*

Who remembers "helmet hair"? A shellac layer of hairspray held an otherwise breezy-looking hairstyle in place. Head moves, hair does not. We now embrace movement in hairstyles and we can do the same with our bodies. Bending, stretching, reaching, are all things we need to do and should do more often for optimal circulation and lymph drainage. And, yes, breasts should move side to side, bunch up and stretch out, too.

As we explore the lymphatic system we are building our understanding of the extracellular matrix, the interstitial fluid, and the fascia as well.

The lymphatic system is one of our cleaning filters. The liver, lungs, and kidneys also perform filtering functions. Most of us are aware of lymph nodes, tiny bean-shaped components of the lymphatic system. Felt easily along the sides of the neck and behind the ears, lymph nodes can enlarge or be tender when clearing toxins or infection from an area like a cold or sore throat.

Lymph nodes are one part of the lymphatic system. Packed with hungry white blood cells called macrophages the nodes are fed by a network of soft tubules, the lymphatic vessels. This network of lymph vessels and lymph nodes collects and pre-filters debris in the interstitial fluid before carrying it back to the heart. There the fluid re-enters the bloodstream for further processing and elimination by the organs.

Snug bras and other tight, restrictive clothing feel a lot like scar tissue to me. My hands pick up a stasis of fluid or stagnation with spandex shapers, underwire bras, and bands. It feels something like extra stiff gelatin. "Jell-O Jigglers" or "Knox blocks" come to mind. Happy healthy tissue doesn't feel like finger food. Healthy tissue has a soft, bouncy texture and fine vibration. It feels vibrant.

The largest lymph vessel travels from the abdomen to the chest passing through a little opening in the diaphragm. This thoracic duct receives fluid from both legs, the pelvis, and the abdomen. It transports lymph upward staying close to the spine until it reaches the left side of the neck, near the cute little collarbone dip. Here it makes a hairpin loop through the fascia of the hollow behind the collarbone and re-enters the chest, destined for the heart. A smaller lymph vessel tucks under the right collarbone to serve the right arm, chest, and right half of the head. Why did I take extra care to share this with you? Any impairment to alignment, congestion, or scarring along this lymphatic path from both legs, pelvis, trunk, and the left half of the head disrupts the lymphatic flow!

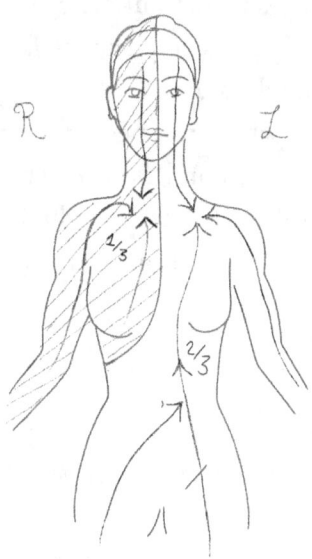

Figure 8.8: Pathways of the Right and Left Thoracic Lymphatic Flows

Here is an example. An active 47-year-old patient had sought help for persistent swelling in his knee after an ACL, anterior cruciate ligament, repair. It had been over 3 months since the surgery, but the swelling wouldn't budge. Surgery had otherwise been successful and he had faithfully performed physical therapy exercises. He had additionally received oral steroids, prednisone, and steroid injections of cortisone to tame the swelling. These medicines are very strong anti-inflammatory treatments, but the persistent swelling was stronger. Upon examining the patient I saw that his left collarbone was notably misshapen. It had healed jagged and overlapped from a nasty break 30 years earlier. He was treated with osteopathic lymphatic and fascial manipulation. I focused on the collarbone and diaphragms of the body treating with hands-on osteopathy. His knee swelling decreased visibly during treatment despite not treating the "knee" proper. By morning the knee size and mobility were nearly normal. He reported that during his physical therapy appointment that week his surprised therapist examined and exclaimed, "What happened?!"

In short, the ECM, interstitial fluid and lymphatic system perfuse every other tissue and organ system. The fascia provides the structural matrix for these special fluid systems.

You noticed that osteopathic treatment of the patient with knee swelling focused on the diaphragm and clavicle. The body is all one piece! Learn more about the full body effects, including lifting up organs, of the diaphragm right after the star of the show, breast tissue!

Breast tissue

Skin, electromagnetics, fascia, and lymph, you have really learned a lot! Each of these is present in the breast as well. Breast tissue is glandular tissue that develops from a specialized sweat gland (refer to cross-section of skin). The shape of breast tissue is something of a tilted teardrop like an apostrophe or an eighth note if you're musical. It has a circular center with a tail extending toward the armpit. Adipose (fat) tissue fills out breasts to give them their unique shape. Many women comment that when they lose weight the breasts are the first to show it owing to the plumping fat content. Be assured, the breast tissue is still present!

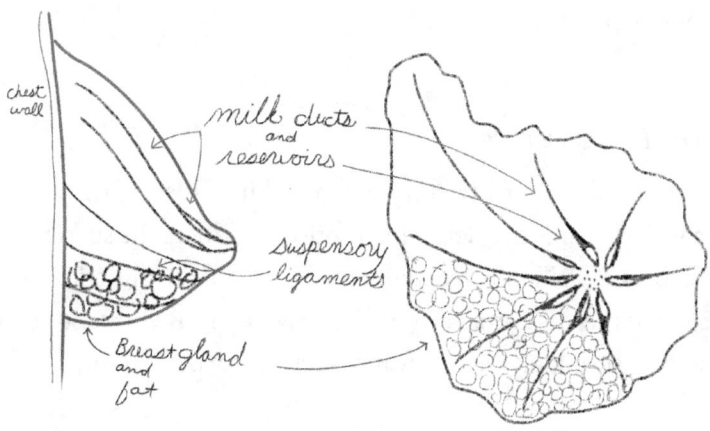

Figure 8.9 Breast Gland Tissue from Side-view and Front-view
Milk ducts converge toward the nipple forming a radial pattern as seen in the "front" illustration. As they near the nipple, the ducts widen into milk reservoirs, and then narrow again to exit the nipple tip. These are the little "doors" or pores mentioned in Chapter 4, The Match-up, earlier.

Breast support and position are dependent on several variables. Two anatomical structures include suspensory ligaments also known as Cooper's ligaments and the transverse septum forming the lower border of the breast.

Cooper's ligaments are fine fibers of collagen attached from inside the skin and anchoring on fascia overlying muscles of the chest wall.

The transverse septum is a thickened tissue that forms the lower border of the breast and is sometimes referred to as the breast root. It defines the position and shape of the base, narrow to wide and closely spaced versus farther apart.

Lymph fluid from interstitial fluid floats and flows through the extra-cellular matrix formed of fascia. And the electrical system supports each cell and tissue. Later, self-care built on the knowledge of anatomy will help you enhance form and function of these tissues.

I have witnessed a reduction in tender cysts, pre-menstrual swelling and breastfeeding mastitis with support of the lymph drainage and optimizing the energetic flow.

Muscles and the diaphragm

Muscles under your bra run your breathing. Ideally, the abdominal diaphragm's doming and flattening motion produces the suction needed to create breath. When the diaphragm is not able to function properly such as when there is a strap around it, accessory muscles assist in moving the ribs and shoulders. This creates suction to pull in air, but not as efficiently.

As the diaphragm contracts it flattens and moves downward creating suction inside the thorax (chest cavity). Air is pulled into airways and lungs, as is blood into the heart to fill for the next heart contraction. And, of course, lymph! Lymphatic fluid is pulled into the chest cavity from the body to rejoin blood circulation.

The diaphragm is a large sheet of muscle tissue. It is attached in a circle all the way around the inside of the ribcage. Attachments reach downward in front to the bottom edge of ribs and in back all the way down to the first and second lumbar vertebra inside your spine.

There are three large openings in this muscular dome for the aorta carrying arterial blood, vena cava carrying venous blood, and esophagus carrying food to the stomach. The largest lymph vessel, thoracic duct, shares a doorway with the aorta. Little slender slits allow for smaller nerves and vessels to pass as well. It reminds me of the St. Louis Arch, "Gateway to the West." There is a lot of traffic here.

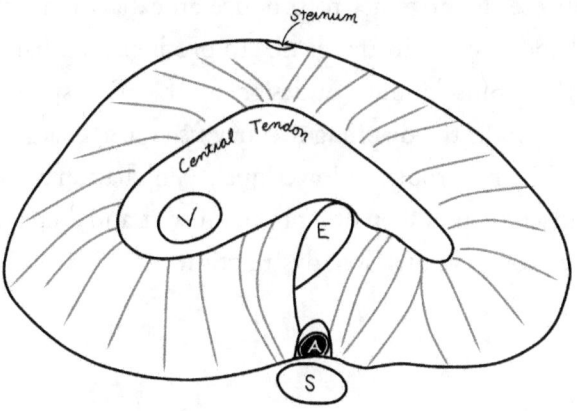

Figure 8.10: Diaphragm from Abdominal View
The thoraco-abdominal diaphragm viewed from below. Structures that pass through the diaphragm are labeled: Vena Cava (V), Esophagus (E), Aorta (A), and Spine (S). Note the direction of the fibers and the loop around the esophagus.

The abdominal diaphragm works in synchrony with the thoracic inlet and pelvic diaphragm. Yes, even the pelvic floor and its function or dysfunction is affected by our breath! The suction vacuum created inside the ribcage by the diaphragm creates "lift" for internal organs. It actually reduces the weight of organs. A liver for example weighs an average of 7 pounds but with lift produced by negative pressure inside the chest, it functionally weighs 3 pounds. This is one reason organs do not end up piled on top of one another in the bottom of the pelvis. The medical term for drooping abdominal organs is "abdominal ptosis." Organ prolapse, such as bladder and uterus, can result from a lack of lift.

Accessory muscles of respiration are engaged when the diaphragm is not functioning optimally. As the diaphragm flattens and lowers, the ribcage naturally widens in all directions - front to back, side to side, and top to bottom. A chest strap stops this natural widening. It forces the use of "accessory" muscles of respiration. These muscles include the intercostal, scalene, and sternocleidomastoid. Intercostal muscles attempt to squeeze ribs together to produce an exhalation, while scalene and sternocleidomastoid lift upper ribs to produce an inhalation. These are hard-working muscles but not designed for 24/7 respiratory use and are not as efficient as the diaphragm. They use more energy and oxygen to work like this and produce a lower quality inhalation and exhalation. Accessory muscles can pull on other neck muscles and even contribute to temporo-mandibular joint, TMJ, dysfunction.

Esophagus

The esophagus deserves special attention due to its relationship to the diaphragm and its association with the dysfunction "GERD" or gastro-esophageal reflux disease. "E" is for esophagus, the muscular tube that moves food from the mouth to the stomach. To reach the stomach it must pass through a small opening in the diaphragm. This diaphragm effectively forms a sphincter, a loop of muscle fibers in this case, to hold food and digestive juices in the stomach and not wash back into the esophagus. What happens when diaphragm motion is restricted, or twisted? It limits the function of the sphincter. Diaphragm dysfunction is a frequent finding in GERD, gastro-esophageal reflux disease. When diaphragm restriction is addressed and treated, reflux symptoms often resolve. Treatment is focused on removing obstacles to health. This could be a bra band or belt or offering osteopathic treatment to balance the tissue.

The pelvic floor and other diaphragms

Ready, ladies? What comes with age-related changes and rhymes with "Depends"? Pelvic floor *dys*function. It doesn't rhyme. And for thousands of women, it's not funny. Muscles of the pelvic floor form slings and sphincters woven into a supportive basket. This basket floor at the bottom of the trunk holds up organs, regulates the passage of urine and feces, and can accommodate the birth of a child. That is pretty impressive. When it is unable to perform its functions, bladder leakage, urinary incontinence, organ prolapse (organs falling out through the urethra, vagina, or rectum), and painful intercourse are just a few of the day-to-day sufferings that result.

That sounds awful, but how did this get in the "bra book"?

By now, you have seen the interrelationship of pieces to the whole, form to function. In the section on thoracic diaphragm, we saw the important role of providing negative pressure (suction) inside the ribcage to "hold up" abdominal organs. This negative pressure also holds up pelvic organs including bladder and uterus. Men have pelvic floors, too. Dysfunction can urinary and defecation problems for them, as well as sexual dysfunction.

There are several views of thought regarding causes of pelvic floor dysfunction. The three most commonly recognized are 1. prior injury, 2. muscles being too weak, and 3. muscles that are too strong. Of course, this is a simplification and we will soon see the inter-relationships of these models.

Most vaginal childbirth constitutes an injury to the perineum and pelvic floor. Giving birth, whether recent or not, is the most widely mentioned cause of pelvic floor dysfunction in medical literature. All childbirth requires a prior condition, pregnancy! And pregnancy causes a multitude of changes to the anatomy and physiology of the mother including crowding of lungs and abdominal organs, impairing the motion of the thoracic diaphragm, and softening all of the connective tissue through hormonal changes.

The issue of muscle weakness has been addressed with Kegel's exercises for many years. However, weakness can also be caused by prior injury and a need to retrain nerves or address fascial strain. "Muscles too strong" is another way to say "tense." The muscles are unable to relax, so they are unable to receive optimal nerve and blood flow. Injury can result in weakness and tension in the same tissue!

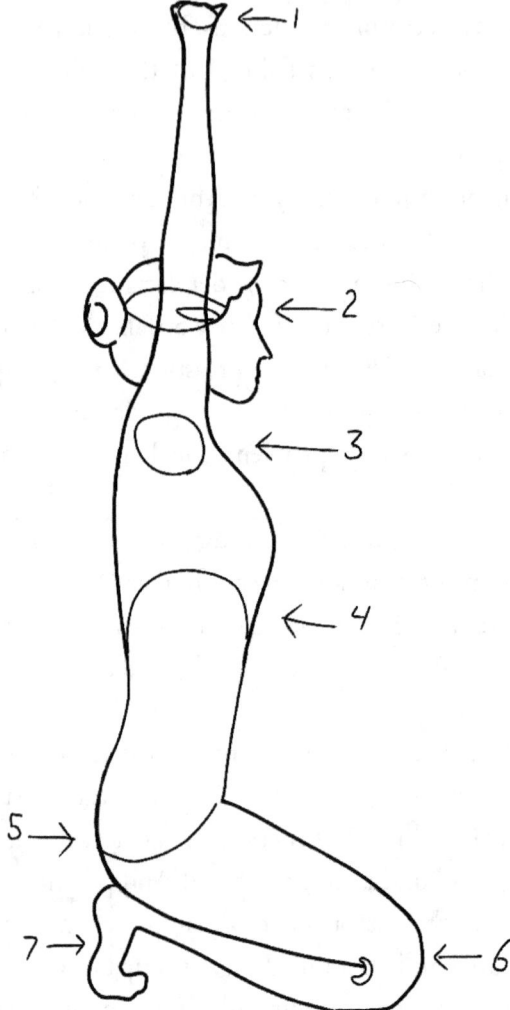

Figure 8.11: Diaphragms of the Body Stacked Like a Tall Drum
From the hands to the feet multiple diaphragms move in synchrony. The tentorium is inside the skull. The thoracic inlet at the top of the rib cage. The abdominal diaphragm at the bottom of the ribs separates the heart and lungs from the digestive organs. The pelvic diaphragm is a sling formed by muscles of the pelvic floor.

Still, why include this in a book about bras?

Ah ha! We must venture back to the ribcage with beautiful spongy air-filled sacs and the thoracic diaphragm's ability to create suction, like a piston. As the diaphragm descends, widening and flattening, it creates a vacuum for air to enter lungs. Prior injury to lungs can leave scarred areas or lung tissue that does not have the same recoil. Scars decrease the ability to make this suction force, and the liver now weighs 7 pounds again, or at least a lot more than it did with spongy, elastic lungs and a freely moving diaphragm. What do a bra band and shoulder straps feel like to an osteopath's hands? It feels like scar tissue. Scar tissue texture feels rigid under my touch. It does not have much liquid or flow sensation. And it restricts movement.

Without the aid of suction to provide lift the liver weighs 7 pounds again as well as other organs, stomach, spleen, kidneys, intestines, uterus, and bladder. The full weight of these organs places additional stress on the delicate balance of the pelvic floor.

There are other diaphragms, sheets of tissue stretched across the body that act a bit like a drum skin. The top of the trunk is capped by the thoracic inlet. Going up even further, inside the head we have tough layers lining the skull and forming slings to support brain tissue. To finish the set we go out to the palms of the hands and soles of the feet to find a peripheral set of diaphragms. If we imagine these four central drum skins stacked vertically and the hands up, feet down we have a column of vibration unifying the movement of a multilayered drum. Music moves the fluid.

Bones and joints

My second-grade teacher had a stand-up easel at the front of the classroom for lessons. One day it was covered with sheets of cellophane displaying a series of illustrations of the human body. It was a lift-the-flap game. First, we peeled off the top layer, a drawing of skin, to see what was under it. Next, we uncovered muscles, organs appeared, and finally, we were down to the picture of a skeleton. Just like Halloween! My teacher summarized the lesson with this graphic mental image: "Without bones, you would be a pile of mush -- just a blob on the floor. Bones are what hold us up."

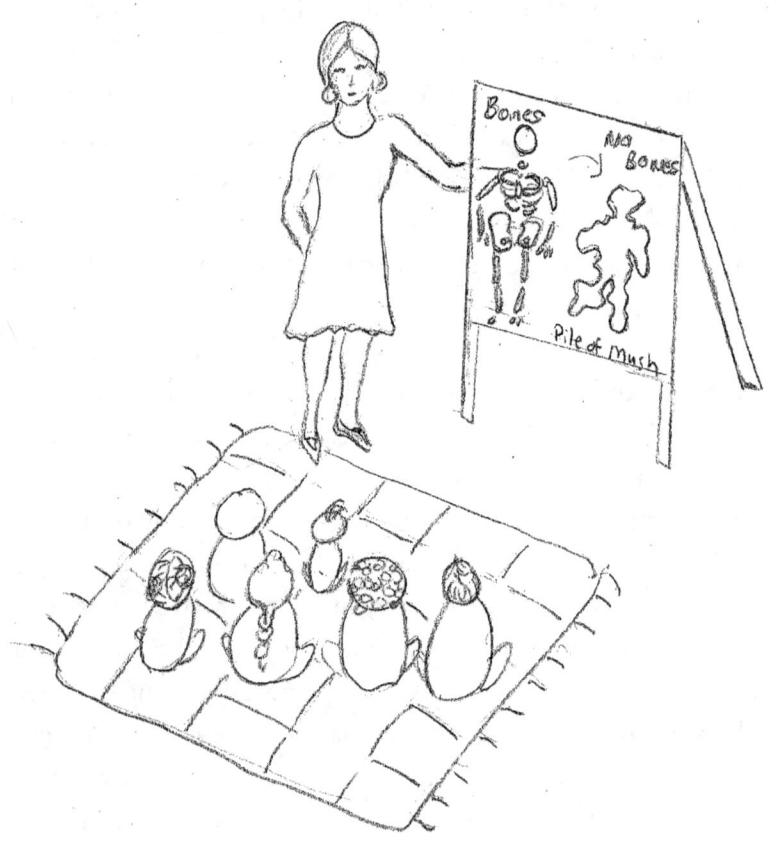

Figure 8.12: Author's First Anatomy Class, 2nd Grade
The function of bones was misrepresented in my early anatomy training, leading one to believe that without bones we would just be a pile of mush on the floor. Although bones contribute to structure, the statement was not entirely true.

I want to believe she believed this. But it isn't true. Tensegrity holds us up. Physics holds us up, and qi holds parts in place.

Imagine your bones. Finger bones, ribs, spine, forehead. How do we describe them? Hard and bony! When you think of bone do you imagine cooked bones left on your plate after dinner? White, dried out, and brittle? Or do you imagine a living tissue like a tiny sapling in the woods bending in the breeze? Bone cells and matrix form a dense but malleable tissue. Living bone is as much like dead bone as a tree sapling is like a table leg! A young tree can be molded and shaped as it grows, and so can a young ribcage. Bones respond and reshape throughout our lives, giving us a chance to prevent and correct injury.

Our bones are broken down and rebuilt continuously thanks to special bone cells called osteoclasts and osteoblasts. Wolff's Law states that new bone is laid down in lines of stress. You can imagine a stress line by bending a twig and noticing where it gives first. Bone is shaped and reshaped according to the pressure on it. It explains why weight-bearing bones develop into thicker denser bones than non-weight-bearing bones. Since we are continually breaking down old bone and making new bone it also means we can change the future shape of our skeleton.

I would often point out to women on the treatment table the dip in their ribs at the level of the bra band or underwire. Just below that space is a flare-outward of the ribs above the abdomen. Most were surprised to feel this dip and flare. I suggested they go home, take a look at the guys in their home, and note the absence of dips in their ribcages. There may be changes that feel like dents and bumps from healed rib fractures. (The guys have their own risks of rib deformation from more frequent impact injuries!) The good news is bone is living tissue and can re-mold when impediments are removed.

There is a special series of joints to know. The costovertebral joint makes its home up and down both sides of the spine from base of the neck to lower back. This is the hinge that allows the ribs to swing up and down with the breath. Just in front of it is a lump of nerve tissue, a sympathetic ganglion, which is responsible for carrying fight or flight or freeze information to our organs. These sympathetic nervous system ganglia are soothed by the rhythmic motion of breath and activated by lack of breathing or mechanical pressure. Consider how a snug bra strap applies pressure to these nerves and constricts the breath itself.

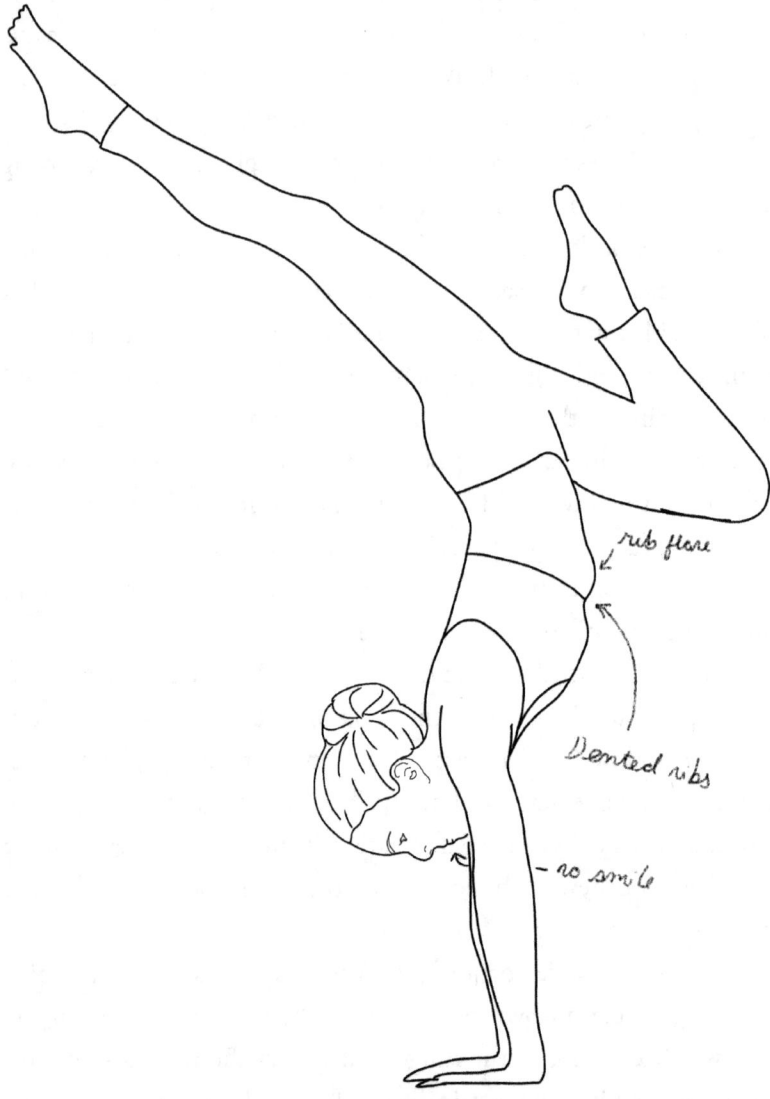

Figure 8.13A: Yoga Ribcage with Bra-band Deformity
Ribcage deformed by tight bra band, note the rib-flare and lack of smile.

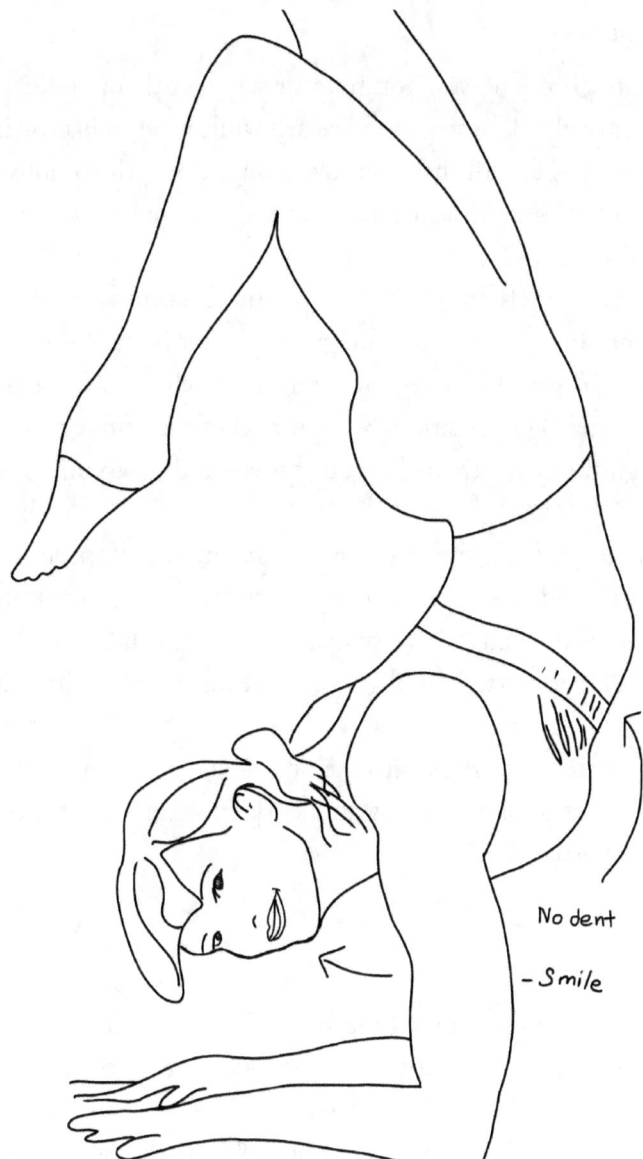

Figure 8.13B: Happy Yoga Ribcage
Ribcage in natural shape, note the soft wrinkles in the clothing and wide, soft band.

Take a full breath now. Is it relaxing? Is it tight and anxious? Check if your ribs expand side to side and front to back or if your shoulders are riding up to create space for air.

Spinal cord and nerves

Ah, now we reach the nerves. You have already met them beside the spine. Nerves form right alongside blood vessels while we are still growing inside mom's womb. Each rib has a groove along its length to house a nerve, artery, and vein bundle as it travels from the spine in back to the front of the body.

The spinal cord travels from brain down the back in a protective spinal canal formed in vertebra. The cord gives off nerve branches to serve levels of the body. These branches carry sensory (feeling) information and motor (movement) information. Some branches perform regulatory function through the sympathetic nervous system and parasympathetic nervous system.

Sympathetic nerves from the bra-strap area, thoracic 5-9 specifically, innervate the gallbladder, stomach, liver, pancreas, spleen, and upper small intestine. Pressure can irritate sympathetic nerves and keep these organs in a state of high alert: fight, flight or freeze instead of a calm state: rest and digest.

Our organs love to support us with their rest and digest calm state. In the following sections we'll meet a few and let them share their stories as I experienced them with patients.

Lungs

This is a good time for a breathing break. What you have learned above has been a lot of new anatomy and physiology. So, go ahead, get up and reach, shake, and blow off some tension. We'll visit the lungs to learn about these unique delicate organs of pink chiffon that support our life's breath!

Healthy lung tissue is pink and spongy due to its meshwork of minute blood vessels lining tiny air sacs. The very stretchy elastic tissue forms airways, bronchi, which branch into smaller and smaller bronchioles, ending in tiny sacs called alveoli. In these nearly 500 million alveoli is where oxygen and carbon dioxide exchange and respiration occurs. Toxins and cellular waste products are also released with respiration. Lungs are one of the body's organs of detoxification like the liver, kidneys, and skin.

In traditional Chinese medicine (TCM), lungs are viewed as the governor over its territory. Each organ governs an emotion, a season, an element, and more. Lungs are chief governor over the emotion of grief, the season of autumn, and the metal element. I imagine the metal element as tendrils of pure gold infused with the strength of steel.

In all disciplines of health I have had the opportunity to study, breathing comes foremost. Ancient systems of health and wellness such as Ayurveda/yoga and TCM dedicate volumes of material to teaching daily breathing practices. Western medicine places high importance on ABC's, airway, breathing, and circulation for emergency interventions. Daily breathing practice keeps the instrument of the body well-tuned.

It is thrilling to work with a patient and have the perception of organs communicating their messages. Unprocessed or "stuck," emotions tend to stay in their governor organ. An emotional insult to lungs such as a great loss or grief can get stuck and result in airway inflammation, congestion, or cough as the governor works to clear the emotion. Once processed, emotions travel to the abdominal diaphragm for storage until they can pass to intestines and on out of the body. This is such a fascinating model of health. More importantly, it gives us a practical application for optimal breathing and the need for full expansion of the diaphragm.

A baseline of healthy breathing and circulation allows the emotional body to process and assimilate emotions. Optimal breathing keeps the body and mind in balance.

Lungs rely on the muscular diaphragm to create the space and suction needed to fully stretch the lungs to take in air and make an efficient exchange with the blood in the capillaries. If the diaphragm is tight and restricted or weak and tired, the "accessory muscles of respiration" take over. These are muscles in the neck and between the ribs. Using these muscles signals to the brain a state of panic. More interestingly, *when a tight band is placed around the chest it inhibits the diaphragm from descending and widening out, which consequently activates the accessory muscles and sympathetic nervous system.*

Each beat of the heart supplies the meshwork of lungs with venous blood through the pulmonary artery. Breath revitalizes this blood with oxygen and light photons. It returns to the heart until the next beat to be carried out to the body through the aorta.

Heart

The Emperor of organs in TCM is the Heart! Of course it is, you say, but I always wondered if Western medicine would have chosen the brain. We really like things to make sense. But, alas, "brain" in TCM roughly translates to "sea of marrow" and doesn't evoke images of logic.

As Emperor, Heart overseas the other organs and emotions while directly processing joy and sadness. I think of "a heart full of joy" as the goal. The human heart also perceives and processes all types of information. And, of course, its main collaborator is the brain. This heart-brain connection was present before birth. The physical position of the head and heart were folded together when we were in our embryo form.

Fascinating studies have shown that the heart responds to a stimulus before the brain has awareness. This was measured by placing both EEG and EKG on volunteers. While subject's eyes were closed, different images were placed in front of the participant. The EKG tracing showed the heart responding before the brain EEG. If you have ever awoken with a strong sensation in your chest, your heart, either positive or negative, only to discover a coinciding event later, you'll understand what I'm referring to here. The electrical system of the heart is so strong it radiates energy that can be *measured* several feet from the body.

The HeartMath Institute shares more research regarding the heart's energy field. This is measured and recorded easily with an EKG machine, a common medical test to assess the health of heart function by tracing its electrical conduction.

Heart rate variability (HRV) has in recent years come to the forefront in biofeedback medicine. The idea is that a bit of variation between heartbeats is a physiologic marker of being in a relaxed healthy, healing, state. With phone apps and home equipment available online, a person can follow their own HRV. The variability reflects the heart's response to internal and external environments. I think of the phrase "a peaceful state of mind." Now we know it is a peaceful state of *heart and mind* that is associated with well-being.

At a conference in 2014, I visited with a medical school classmate. For many years, she had practiced as a radiologist interpreting X-ray, ultrasound, CAT scan, and MRI images. Shifting gears in her career, she was now in a post-graduate program for osteopathic manipulative medicine. For her original research to complete the program, she had performed an MRI on herself *with* and *without* wearing a bra. She then *measured the deformity* of her heart and lungs when wearing a bra as compared to when she was not. Wow. She had measured and confirmed what my hands perceived daily in the office; a restriction in patients' hearts.

Additionally, I was sensing "quietness" in people's hearts. Some were peaceful. Some were not. As I became more attuned I realized some sensations of what initially seemed to be "quietness" were actually apathy, a state of not feeling and not expressing. The sensation is something like being asleep or resigned. The communication within the body from the heart to the tissues was not optimal. Interestingly, when I delicately mentioned this to patients, they shared that their relationships felt similar, lacking in *something not easily defined*. "Communication of joy?" I wondered silently.

An open heart means many different things to different people and at different times. What I have noticed consistently is that as the energy of the heart expands and the breath flows, such as after a treatment, it is counterproductive to put the chest wall back into a brace that fit the former apathetic condition.

The heart forms a beautiful central complex within the chest. The largest artery, aorta, and largest vein (vena cava) join the heart directly. A meshwork of nerve fibers travels along the blood vessels. And our friends, the lymph vessels and nodes coalesce in a balance point at the center of our chests.

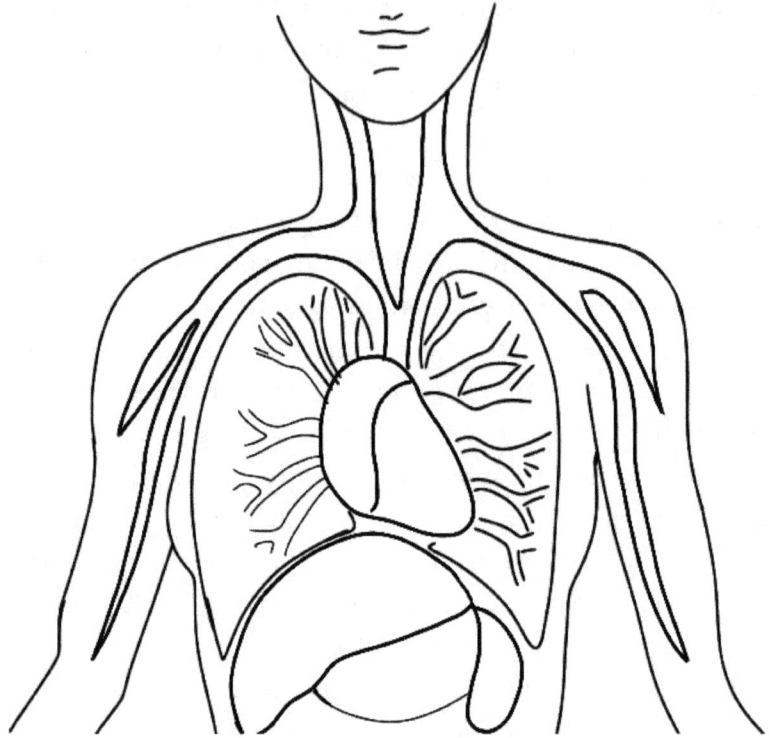

Figure 8.14: Central Heart Balance Point

Liver and gallbladder

Grrr, grrr, says the liver. Not really, but it is the chief governor over the emotion of anger. Anger translates to other words, too, such as frustration and irritation. It includes the little pokey nudges that keep us from feeling too comfortable when something really needs to change. Anger stokes the fire (heart element in TCM) with wood (liver element) to give us motivation. A healthy liver can process anger in all these forms, allowing the emotion to process and pass when it is no longer needed.

What happens with a congested liver? For physicians, patients are our teachers. And, "conversations" with the liver taught me many causes of congestion and inflammation. The organ as a whole may be dealing with a challenge in alignment from an injury or intra-abdominal scars. Its cells may be strained under a load of toxins to breakdown such as medication, alcohol or environmental toxins. Finally, the electrical or subtle energy system could be challenged with a difficult situation at home or on the news. Usually, there was a factor from each. I also found that in listening to the organ it would give its own blueprint for healing. This guided treatment allowed the liver to begin to move more functionally on its own axis, receive fresh nourishing blood and release processed physical toxins with greater ease. Addressing and releasing stuck emotion was a key player in health and integration. In all the livers I've listened to, none requested a restrictive band around the chest. But, instead the organ asked for the diaphragm to be optimized to create natural motion needed for the liver and gallbladder to function.

Where do you find a talking liver? Place your hands on the front of your chest, below the breasts and on the ribs. The liver sits deep to the ribs under your right hand. It is a large solid wedge-shaped organ that fills space from front to back and from the right side to just a bit past center in front. It weighs about 7 pounds. Wow, but get this, as I mentioned earlier, due to the suction force from the inside of the ribcage above the diaphragm, the organ's functional weight is reduced by a third or more. The result is the liver feeling like 3 pounds. This starts to explain why our organs don't all ball up in the bottom of our bellies and fall out. It also gives one possibility as to what the problem is when organs *do* try to fall out. As previously mentioned, this is called prolapse and can happen with bottom-end organs such as the bladder, uterus, or rectum.

According to our Western, Cartesian, model of medicine, wherein the sum of the parts makes up the "whole," the liver is part of the digestive system. Indeed, it produces and secretes bile stored in the gallbladder. Bile flows into the small intestine after a meal to help break down fats in food. But the liver is also an organ of protein production, immune function, and detoxification.

Adding the model of TCM to our tool bag reveals another tidbit. The liver meridian, which flows from the great toe up the inner leg, circles the groin and continues up to the lower ribcage, has a surprising effect on libido and sexual function -- a positive one. Several patients happily confided that bedroom time had greatly improved after finding and fixing their liver meridian.

Spleen and pancreas - digestion and metabolism - blood sugar regulation

Learning about the spleen and pancreas in my Western education focused on two very different organs and purposes. The spleen, a dense solid structure, provided some filtering of blood, specifically red blood cells and produced white blood cells to combat bacterial infection. The pancreas was an organ of the digestive system secreting enzymes, amylase and lipase, to digest carbohydrates and fats. It also was an organ of the endocrine system secreting insulin a hormone to regulate blood sugar. The spleen and pancreas shared some blood vessels to the liver but that was as far as the Cartesian model went for me. Needless to say, I was surprised to see the spleen and pancreas "lumped together" in TCM studies. It provided a new lens through which to view connections in health.

Despite all the functions of the spleen, we can actually survive without one. But, not having a spleen leaves someone vulnerable to bacterial infections. The pancreas is more critical to survival and we need to have at least part of it available and functioning.

Are you ready to locate your spleen and pancreas?

Go back to the liver exercise with hands placed on the lower ribs in front. The spleen is deep to your left hand this time. Now, move your right hand to the upper part of your soft belly, where ribs come to meet in the center like an upside-down "V." The pancreas is deep to your hand behind the stomach. Later I will describe how to use neurolymphatic points for self-care and healing. The spleen/pancreas reflex point, a great re-set button, is on the side of the ribs over the spleen on the left, and the liver on the right.

The interesting thing about the Spleen-Pancreas complex in TCM is that it makes and stores the qi used from day to day. In this way, it relates to our western physiology of the parasympathetic nervous system, the "rest and digest" part of our autonomic nervous system. Spleen meridian is paired with its opposite, the Triple Warmer meridian. Triple Warmer activates with flight or fright like our sympathetic nervous system. I find it fun to see the different models of health merge. No model is perfect. I say to my students, "If your findings (history and physical exam) and solution (treatment plan) don't produce the desired result, get a new model!" This is how the spleen, a digestive organ in the "take it or leave it" section of my surgery training, suddenly became part of the nervous system.

If you do not have a spleen, from whatever cause, do not fret. All is not lost. When I work with people who have had an organ removed the energetic blueprint of it is still present. Having the physical organ is very useful but it is not everything. The energetic blueprint of the organ still has a presence and potency.

Kidneys

Por fin! We meet the kidneys. Why, you ask? Aren't they somewhere down in your back? Can you live without them? No. With just one kidney, yes, you can survive, but we have two kidneys for a reason. As with other paired organs, lungs and gonads, with two kidneys there is a back-up.

Let's first locate our own kidneys and then look at why they have anything to do with bras. This time, place your hands on either side of your waist at about belly button level. Turn your hands so the fingers wrap around your back and your thumbs are in front. Your fingers will be lying over the more firm-feeling ribs versus the thumb on the soft belly. If you have a wider waist, move your whole hand back around toward your spine, close to the midline. Your kidneys are "kidney-bean shaped" dense, solid organs about the size of your fists. They lie under the ribs in back and reach below the rib line a few centimeters. How far up or down they are depends on whether you are inhaling or exhaling and how you are breathing. Ideally, your kidneys will move up and down a good 6 cm with each breath, tucking way up under the ribs and descending below them. Our lungs and diaphragm make this motion possible. The kidneys also make a gentle rotation inward and outward as they go, forming a link to breath, bra, and body.

Our paired kidneys are supplied with nutrient-rich blood by renal arteries. They filter our blood of impurities and help break down chemicals for them to be passed out of the body with water. This watery product is urine flowing through ureters into the bladder. The urethra then carries the urine through the pelvic floor opening and out of the body. Amazing. Kidneys are related to flow of breath, purity of blood, expansion of lungs and movement of thoracic and pelvic diaphragms!

Kidneys are host to two special organs called adrenal glands. The Latin word for kidney is *renal*. The "ad" renal is a soft little gland that sits on top of the kidney itself. A plethora of hormones are produced here, including adrenaline, cortisol, estrogen, progesterone, testosterone, and DHEA. These hormones are major players in our level of health and vitality. In recent years, I have been drawn to the number of articles related to a phenomenon called "adrenal fatigue" and even more articles regarding chronic anxiety due to fight-or-fight response. Both are built on the premise of over-activation of the adrenal hormones due to chronic stress.

Traditional Chinese medicine adds dimension with the concept of primordial qi stored in kidneys. The adrenal gland is combined with kidney in terms of function and treatment. In this model, primordial qi is the energy, the life force, you were born with. Primordial qi is also referred to as kidney qi. It is something like a battery with a certain amount of charge. The charge is used up over a lifetime at varying rates and when it's gone so is our physical life. Needless to say, preserving kidney qi is quite important in this model. In the TCM model the kidney and kidney meridian govern the emotion of fear. This brings us back to the fight, flight, or freeze response produced by the adrenal glands. Chronic stress response involving the release of adrenaline and cortisol is considered deleterious in both models of medicine. In all models of health and medicine a peaceful, calm state is healing.

Now that we know what's between bra cups and bra backs. Let's look at some examples and see how things size up.

III

Outfitting

9

Making the Most of What We Have

You've decided it is in your best interest to wear a bra for specific occasions whether it be the workplace or comfort for exercise. Let's look at how to use a bra to your best advantage. How can you maximize the benefits while wearing one and minimize the side effects? In Chapters 9 and 10 we will review common bra styles available off the rack today. After determining the goals to be met for a particular bra-wearing activity, I'll help guide your thought process to narrow the selection. Finally, we meet your closet and I'll share some DIY alterations to fine-tune your new and old selections. The goal to be met here is to become confident enough to ignore the tag size and trust your own body and tape measure. We can avoid the Emperor's New Clothes folly with confidence and common sense.

The following is a step into the language of lingerie. These are words you may encounter while shopping for bras or patterns to make your own. Having a working knowledge of the terms will help you match your goals and girls. Later, in Chapter 11, we will look at braless options such as tanks and camisoles, as well as clothing styles to complement braless by choice and not attract unwelcome attention.

Cup

Full cup: A full cup is designed to cover the entire breast from armpit across to the breastbone. This style is the most supportive and easiest on breast tissue by avoiding lines of pressure on the tissue but may peek out under a shirt with a lower neckline.

Demi-cup: Part of the upper cup has been removed in a demi-cup to reveal more breast. It does not cover as close to the breastbone.

Balconette: About half coverage in a balconette, the upper edge of the cup is cut horizontally like a balcony with just the nipple covered and the breast spilling out. These are often associated with a bustier or corset bra padded, push-up, and lacey.

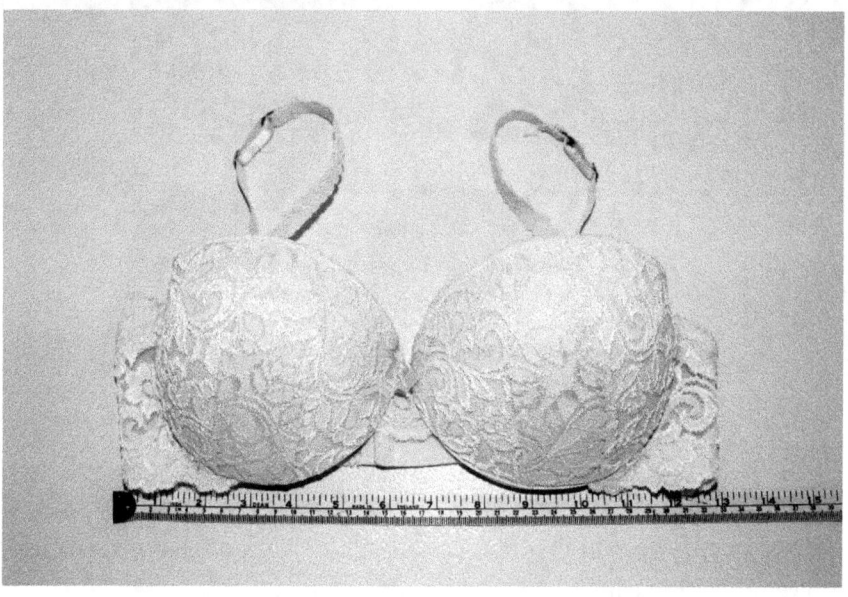

Figure 9.1: Underwire Bra Exhibiting Multiple Characteristics
This underwire, push-up and padded confection has balconette-styled cups. It is also convertible to a single strap, cross-back or strapless bra.

Underwire: Underwire refers to an actual metal wire or a hard plastic C-shape that is tunneled into a casing sewn around the bottom and side of the cup.

Wire free: With no actual metal or plastic in the casing, "wire free" is generally a good term to look for while shopping. But, be aware, if it arrives and *feels* like a wire, treat it like one. I once ordered a wire free bra online to have it arrive with a thick padded foam cup heat fused at the lower edge into a rigid structure (aka underwire).

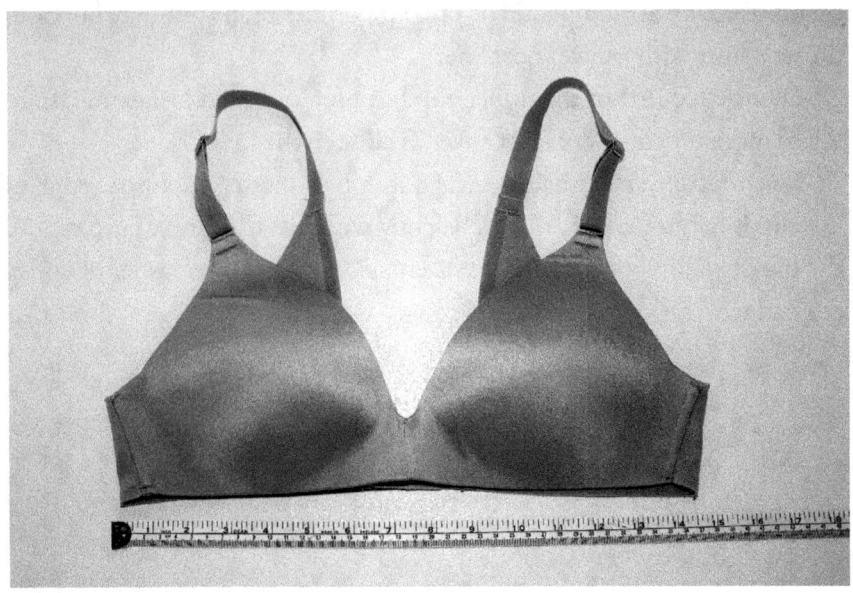

Figure 9.2: Wire free T-shirt Bra with Leotard Styling Back.
The leotard styling of the straps to the back band allows the straps to come closer together in back reducing the incidence of straps falling off the shoulder and better accommodating a bra extender.

Unlined: One layer of fabric over the breast, ranging from sheer to opaque.

Lined: More than one layer. Although padded styles would be considered lined, lined alone often refers to a simple second layer of fabric or polyester fiber batting.

Padded: Thick, even layer of padding throughout the cup. These are thick enough to prevent nipple show-through and are often advertised as adding a cup size.

Push-up: Padded cup with additional thickness in the lower half of the cup to push the breasts up and towards each other to produce cleavage.

Closure

Back hook: Hook and eye closure in the back of the bra typically with 2 or 3 rows of hooks but may be as few as one or up to 5. There are 3 settings of length, tightest, middle, and loosest. The entire range from tight to loose is less than an inch.

Front hook: A metal or plastic clasp between the cups in front. These can be easier to put on and off but, there is no option for customizing the band length.

Pull-over: A one-piece construction that is pulled over the head or in crafty situations stepped into and pulled-up. The step in maneuver protects shoulders from overhead movement. The original JogBra is a pullover style as are some comfort bras and day bras.

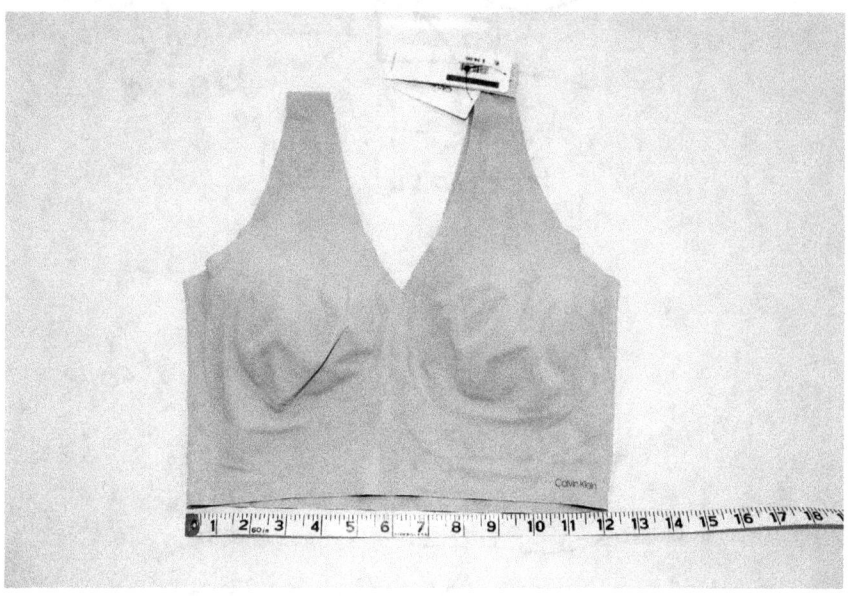

Figure 9.3: Pull-over Comfort Bra Styling with Removable Foam Cups.
This bra is labeled as size XL. Like many styles and models it's actual size is quite small, this one measures 26 inches around the rib cage/bra band.

Sports bra: An athletic bra can come in one of two breast support options: compression or encapsulated. Compression is as it sounds and is meant to flatten the breast tissue down close to the body wall. It works well to immobilize breasts of smaller volume during running and jumping. Encapsulated styles gain strength by separating and encapsulating each breast individually. The best high-impact sports bras I've seen have a high neckline and almost a tank top style to the back and sides.

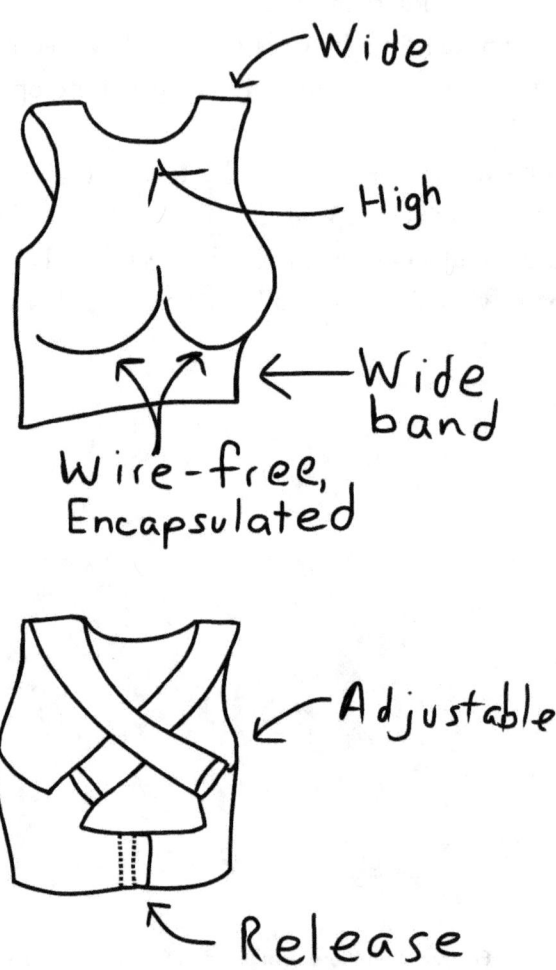

Figure 9.4:
Dr. Coffman's favorite elements are highlighted in this illustration. A high neckline, wide straps and band, wire-free cups and an adjustable quick release back hook.

Strap

Straight: Straight straps go over the shoulders and land perpendicular to the bra band. They are more difficult to keep on the shoulders and even more difficult if a bra extender is added making them farther apart in back.

Curved: A curved design is also called scoop or leotard back. These straps go over the shoulder then begin to curve toward each other as they meet the band. They form the top edge of the band in back and are generally more close-set than the straight straps. Curved straps receive bra extenders better and don't slip as easily.

Racer back: A no-slip solution, the racer back is designed after swimsuits that cut out the area over the shoulder blade for less restriction in motion. The caveat here is to watch for too much tension. Sizing as we know is variable and many, many patients in my office were in a race-back style with excessive pressure over the shoulder and neck area. This pressure affected the nerves from the neck, the muscles, and lymphatics.

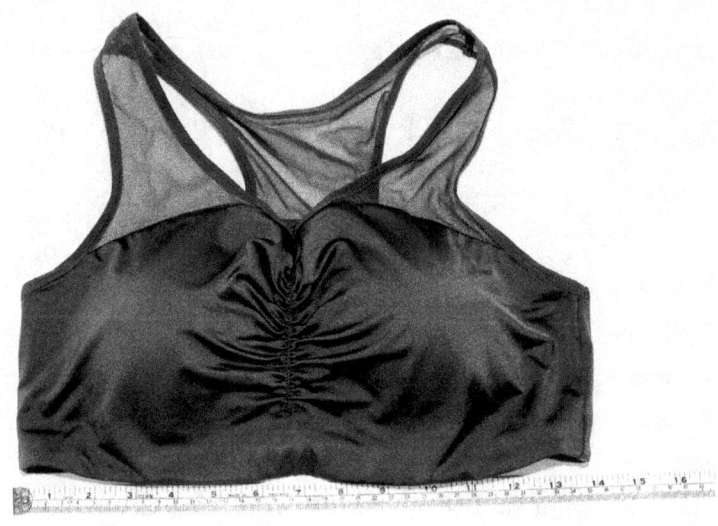

Figure 9.5: Racer Back
This pull-over racerback bra has removable foam cups and a wire free frame. It is shown in an XL despite its resting measurement of 14 inches wide resulting in a 28 inch band.

Specialty

Bralettes: Almost anything goes in styling. Bralettes are generally soft, unlined, and not designed to lift.

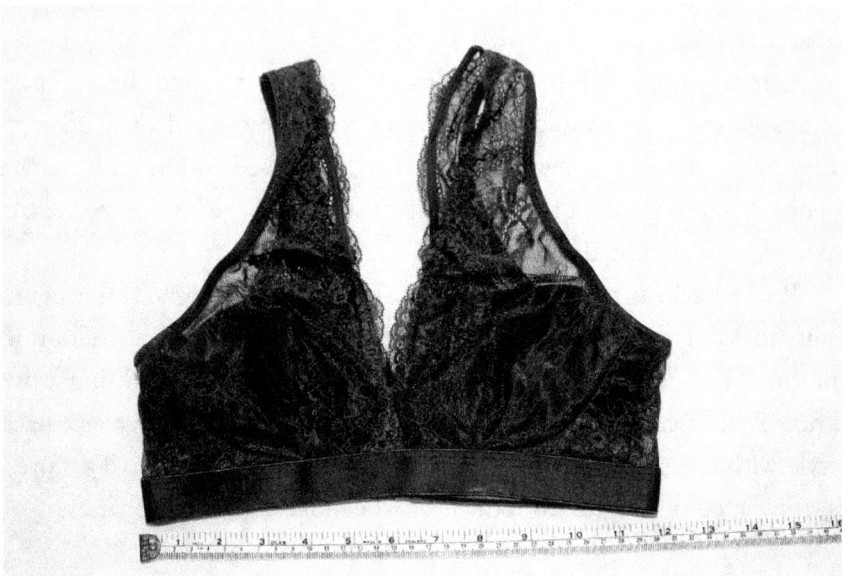

Figure 9.6: Bralette
This bralette has a back-closure and is labeled as size XL.

Strapless: Made for tops and dresses exposing the shoulders.

Backless: Originally designed for backless dresses, I've heard a few people opted for these after reading this book. Designs range from nipple covers to full breast coverage and either stick on with silicone or adhesive. Adhesive has the obvious drawbacks and silicone over milk ducts should be used sparingly.

Pasties: Nipple-cover version of the backless bra.

Post mastectomy with prosthesis pockets: Often traditional in styling but with an extra layer of fabric to make a prosthesis pocket.

Nursing bras: These are built with "trap doors" for access to the nipple. A clasp at the top of the cup or between the cups releases the cup fabric to allow access for breast-feeding.

Orthopedic and posture bras: A combination of upper back brace and breast brace.

You can refer back to this list anytime especially if you decide to look online. For now, start your bra hunt at home and see what is hiding out in your own dresser. Try to name the cup styles, padding, strap style, and so forth. In Chapter 10 you will learn how to refine your desired checklist for best results.

10

What to Look For if Trying Something New

As you can see from the mini glossary, there is a sea of options and marketing. I recommend first to become very clear on what you are looking for in a "bra." You are likely looking for several different items just like footwear. You may even discover there is no particular reason to wear a bra at the moment just like shoes. In which case, you can jump ahead to the next section for no-bra options. The following questions come from reasons women tell me they prefer to wear a bra or something under their clothes. Read on to see what factors may influence your choices.

1. Are you looking for shaping, no nipple show through and fashion-friendly?
2. Do you want to balance out different size breasts or changes from surgery?
3. Are you looking for something to pass the dress code (subtle bra tracks and no nipples) but, you wish it could feel like nothing?
4. Do you need coverage and padding to buffer breasts from small children bumping into you or to provide protection in contact sports?

5. Are you looking for something to prevent chafing/irritation under clothes?
6. Do you want something to absorb sweat under breasts?
7. Do you need to immobilize breasts during bouncy/impact sports? (Hopefully worn very temporarily as we have discussed physiology already!)
8. Are you looking for something beautiful, backless, and strapless for a formal occasion? Can you go au natural? Or do you want to give the illusion of being braless?

Of course, what most women tell me is "Yes, to all of the above! But, it has to be just one bra that can cover it all. Bras are expensive." Yes, they can be. I believe that you really know what is best for your body. Through the resources and pearls in this book, I hope to give you the confidence to know when it is right. I hope these insights inspire creativity! Perhaps you will be inspired to make or re-make your own unders at some point.

Just as in choosing shoes, we want to have the maximum comfort each style or situation can offer. Once you have defined the occasion and purpose consider these shopping points. Realizing as a young friend said, "It's always a compromise."

1. Sister sizing – Measure for a starting point then consider the sister size of that style to have more band length. For example, if a trained bra fitter measures you as a 38C, try starting with a 40B. This will give ribs room to breathe while maintaining a similar cup volume. Begin with sister size 36 D if the opposite is happening in that style and the band is too big and cups too far apart. After considering sister sizes, toss out sizing altogether and use a tape measure to measure the bra. See what matches up best to your own measurements! Genius. This is where I feel the Emperor's New Clothes rings a bell. Don't be fooled by fancy numbers and letters when we can all see there is not enough there to cover the parts. Try all different sizes in a model and check for fit and function. Remember the goal of that bra for a specific activity. Regardless of how much breast immobilization is desired, the band should not create a crease or bulge in your torso and especially not across the breast itself.

	A	B	C	D	E	F	G	H
28	28A	28B	28C	28D	28E	28F	**28G**	28H
30	30A	30B	30C	30D	30E	**30F**	30G	30H
32	32A	32B	32C	32D	**32E**	32F	32G	32H
34	34A	34B	34C	**34D**	34E	34F	34G	34H
36	36A	36B	**36C**	36D	36E	36F	36G	36H
38	38A	**38B**	38C	38D	38E	38F	38G	38H
40	**40A**	40B	40C	40D	40E	40F	40G	40H

Figure 10.1: Sister Sizes Chart
The numbers represent the bra band size and the letters the cup size. The diagonally shaded boxes are examples of sister sizes. Each of these sizes would have similar cup volume.

2. Measure the band – Elastic and spandex want to be their natural size all day, too. As a rule of thumb, measure your own ribcage with a full breath in the area of the bra band. Measure the garment you are considering, and compare. Even super-stretchy pull-over bras can cause a problem due to their "sizing." A medium is usually too small for even a 34-inch bust!

3. Bra extenders – I recommend bra extenders frequently. Being a female physician helps when I want to show a patient how much squeeze is going on with their bra. I ask the patient to unhook the back and let the band come to its resting length. Then I measure the gap formed between the 2 ends to show her. It is usually 2 to 3 inches, but I've seen 6 inches and more! For the 2 to 3-inch span, I recommend an extender or even 2 extenders to give the room needed. Extenders are inexpensive, a few dollars for a package of 2, and can be purchased anywhere sewing notions are sold. I wish I could say they were sold in the bra section. But, alas, we must add to the mystery.

*DIY – A quick color tip from my ballet costume days. Extenders are offered in white and sometimes black. White bra extenders can be tinted to a beige-tan shade by soaking in a cup of plain coffee or tea overnight. Let it dry and rinse. Different brews give differing hues, so enjoy experimenting to find the right shade.

4. Scoop back. Look for styles that offer a leotard-style back, like a scoop where straps curve together to meet instead of being sewn onto the band at right angles. These will accommodate an extender more easily while keeping the straps on the shoulders.

5. Wire free cups. This includes what I call faux wires; plastic strips used in place of wire or heavily fused fabric. I have seen some bras advertised as wire free only to find the cup was "underwired" with multiple layers of fused polyester and polyurethane forming a hard ridge. It is important not to compress the edge of breast tissue or to constrain tissue to edged cups.

*DIY – Many underwire styles can have the casing snipped and the wire removed while retaining the fit of the bra. If the bra fits well to begin with, removing the wire usually retains the fit. Years ago I tried this with one that did *not* fit well. I had nothing to lose. It did not improve. When you are ready to go wire free try this at home. Look inside the bra cup for casing holding the wire. Follow it to the outer edge of the cup and make a tiny snip where you feel the pokey end of the wire. Use small, sharp, pointy scissors to nip. Slide the wire out.

6. Sports Bras – First follow rule of thumb in #1 by measuring yourself and the bra. Try to balance the need for restriction and immobilization versus the need for oxygen in your activity.

7. Metal free – Avoid potential electromagnetic field magnification by opting for wire-free and metal free bras.

8. Toxin free- Choose low or no toxin materials such as organic cotton, wool and linen. Steer clear of polyurethane foam, synthetics, and pesticide sprayed crops of natural materials.

9. Camisoles and tanks with built-in "shelf-bra." Originally, the shelf bra was an extra layer of fabric in the front of the garment secured to side seams. This fabric flap was gathered and secured to an elastic strip that also was sewn to the side seam. This actually works quite well and allows for plenty of rib, heart, and lung health. The shelf-bra does not provide much "lift" or support. It merely gives a bit more coverage and reduces falling out of the bottom of the tank. Today, it's rare to find a front shelf bra. Instead, I find most shelf bras have extended all the way around

inside the tank creating an elastic circumferential band. I'm shocked to see that the size of the elastic band would barely make a garter belt! It's as though the manufacturer kept the elastic length of a front shelf bra and closed it together in back. I've measured 24 inches of elastic on a "medium" shirt. The size chart for the item showed a bust of 36 and waist of 27 for the "medium size." A length of elastic band on the chest that is smaller than the waist measurement is not useful!

*DIY – If you happen upon one of these camisoles or tanks or yoga tops and still really like it, as has happened to me, you can alter it to have elastic only in front. Use a seam-ripper to remove elastic in back and stitch in the elastic to the side seam. This is the more complicated of the DIY solutions I've proposed. A friend with sewing skills can help if you want it to look professional on the inside when you finish. My first one was messy.

As a starting point, Warner's style "Back to Smooth" offers several of the above characteristics and can be viewed online for style and design. Consider a bra extender with it.

Different makers are better at suiting different types of figures. For instance comparing two long-standing companies, Warner and Bali, Warner's offers more styles for those with a slight build while Bali offers several wireless styles for fuller figures.

Returning to the same brand and style you wore for decades may not be successful for two reasons, your body has changed and the bra has changed. Bodies adapt to environmental and physiological changes throughout life. Many of these adaptations also change the shape of the body: skin quality, ribcage shape and size, and breast shape and volume. Bra brands have updated their facilities, materials, and sizing. If your trusty favorite is not a good and functional fit now, these guidelines can help you with new options. But, if you are curious and want suggestions for successful bra free days, read on for a self-paced progress plan.

11

Be Free! Thoughts on how to comfortably reduce or eliminate standard bra wearing

Nipples. There, I said it. Nipples, nipples, nipples. Somewhere during 2020, I was walking along daydreaming when I heard the thought, "If nipples were noses." Hey, don't stop there! I encouraged my train of thought. If nipples were noses, what? Well, if nipples were noses, why would we think they were all the same? Now that noses are all covered with masks when we meet new people, our minds automatically suggest the nose and mouth shapes. But, surprise! I did *not* see that coming.

Fashion is often our cultural shifter with trends going over the line until the line moves. I jokingly told a friend "We will know we've come full circle when bra padding is replaced by nipple enhancers." Fashion trends go to extremes to make a point. They expand boundaries then draw back to a new equilibrium. After a fashion explosion the variation in natural body shapes seem less surprising. Whether it is nipples or noses, big or small, symmetric or not it is just more normal. Imagine bustles under ruffled dresses that got bigger and bigger until someone said "No!"

and pulled on some trousers. I suspect everyone was happy to see a real derriere after years of disguises.

2020 really gave us a chance to explore comfort in clothing at home. I recall a line graph that circulated early that year jokingly displaying the demand for bras, razors, and internet. Bra and razor lines descend across the page while the internet line rises. Later, in the year after lockdown, I overheard several women saying they had headed out for an errand or an outdoor lunch date only to realize they were still braless. I was happy to hear it actually but, not everyone was ready to see it. Social change comes in spurts. So, until then, here are a few fashion and function ideas I learned over the years from lovely patients of all shapes preserving their breath. The goals to be met are ease of breath, fluid circulation, and lymph drainage. In addition, we want the choice of a polished look, one that integrates the body's function and fashion without being distracted by one's choice of underwear.

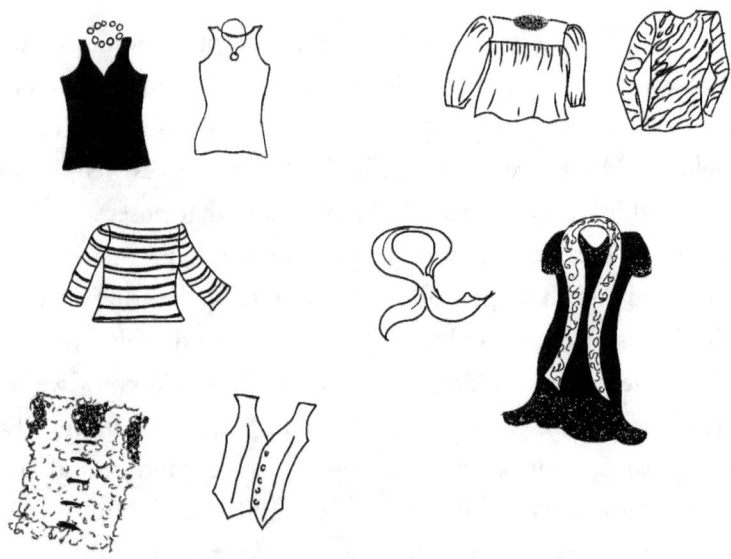

Figure 11.1: Wardrobe Staples for Bra-free Comfort.

Top row: Fitted under layers with varying shapes of necklines, and varying thickness of fabric can replace the bra as first layer. Necklaces help to draw attention upward toward collarbone level.

A gathered blouse with a swing-cut hem provides texture and airflow while a slim-fitting top shines in a pattern of light and dark to mute nipple show-through. Choose outer layers in prints, deeper colors, and textures.

Middle row: Stripes, specifically alternating wide with narrow stripes, offer trompe de l'oeil camouflage. An easy essential to pack and have on hand is a beautiful scarf. Wear it as a piece of art. A scarf will keep you warm in a cool room and divert excess attention from breasts and nipples.

Bottom row: Vests in textured softness or fitted suede add coverage and style.

Getting comfortable with motion and self-image

Great, you went all out and tried it but felt, well, weird. Being comfortable with natural motion of the breasts can take some time. Being confident with self-image may be a process for some women as well. Pace yourself by adding a few of these tips to your daily routine. The small changes can help with adjustment and help you notice the positive results in health. Practice makes perfect, so practice at home and always remember your best posture.

Start with your pajamas. Sleep time is your personal time. Try a natural fiber such as cotton, linen, silk, or wool in a loose fit for both top and bottom. Be aware of restrictive elastic in the waistband, too. You may even discover your sleep is more refreshing!

During the day release the back hook closure of your standard bra as often as possible. You can add bra extenders to decrease tension while keeping up appearances in front. Shoulder straps will feel looser with an extender in the band. You may need to adjust them.

When you are ready for the next step, try a close-fitting, not snug or squeezing, camisole or tank. It should have no shelf bra due to undersized elastic bands. If it does, just clip out the elastic in back of the band.

Eventually, work toward looser undershirts with some air flow available, where fabric does not stick to skin.

To ease into more freedom for exercise activities, remember to size up 2 or 3 generic sizes from the suggested sports bra size. For instance, if your measurements fall into the Medium section, start with an XL. Use real measurements for yourself and the bra. In other words, measure yourself and the garment to see if they match. Disregard the label's numbers.

To control excess movement during high-impact exercise add height to the bra. Controlling the upward bounce can reduce the need for compression in circumference, allowing your heart and lungs better space to function.

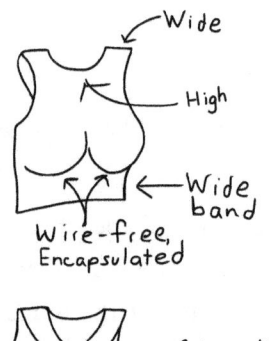

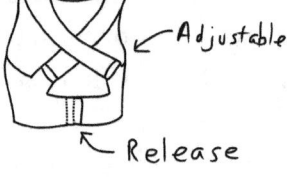

Figure 11.2 High-Impact Activity Brace
The high-impact activity brace illustrates my choice of elements that make up a healthier option for temporarily bracing breasts during exercise.

A high neckline covers the whole bosom up to the clavicles. This reduces the upward motion resulting in less bounce. When breasts go up they must come down. Stop the upward motion before it starts. There is no visible cleavage in this design therefore no "popping out". Note the non-negotiable "release-valve" in back for respiration.

Remember to remove a snug compression-style bra as soon as possible after high-impact exercise is completed. Chapter 12 will give you more encouragement to remove tight bands!

12

Tight Bands, No!

Master Chiao is surveying the room. Headbands, belts, "arch" support socks, memory yarn hosiery, and wristwatches cannot escape his gaze. He approaches, bows, bows again while tapping the offending object. Smile, tap, tap, bow, smile. Poof, it's gone. A tap, tap here and a tap, tap there, he backs to the center of the room to address the class. The hands wave back and forth in a gesture of boundary. "Tight bands. No." His bright black eyes scan our faces for understanding. Satisfied, he nods approval. Class begins.

Good morning, class! Today we will learn to look for the dangers of circumferential bands beginning with the head. Starting soon after birth, hairless babies are often adorned with stretchy ornamental headbands. Baby girls are the subject of flowered headbands and baby boys with tight ball caps. These are to be discouraged on the spot! Babies' brains are growing at a surprising rate every day. A baby's skull made of membrane and cartilage is forming fast as well.

Headbands restrict both growth and inherent motion of the skull and brain tissue. As the head grows rapidly it searches for available areas of growth even if it is not optimal. Have you ever seen a square watermelon? They exist. The little watermelon bud is placed in a box as it grows. It grows and grows to fill every corner of the square box because it is restricted from growing into its oval shape. Nature's design is best in the long run.

Cranial nerves of a human baby can be easily compressed. These are nerves coming directly from the brain to the body (versus from the spinal cord to the body). These nerves exit the skull through openings in the cartilaginous base. Cranial nerves are vitally important to survival. They support feeding (cranial nerves V and VII), swallowing (cranial nerves IX, X, and XII), and digestion and absorption (cranial nerve X, the vagus nerve). The vagus nerve supplies the calming influence that allows baby to bond with their environment. It calms the breath and heart rate helping them to sleep well. The vagus nerve continues these functions at every age! Some indications of cranial dysfunction impairing the nerves are irritability, colic, spitting up, GERD, and feeding difficulties with latch.

Headbands continue through life sometimes in subtle forms such as glasses perched on top like a tiara or plastic headbands shaped like C-clamps. Tight hats and ball caps can also cause cranial dysfunction by compressing the sutures or the base of the skull.

Even more subtle culprits are oral appliances, braces, and eyeglasses. I have treated patients, alongside orthodontist, for many years, to help maintain cranial and full body function during orthodontic treatment. Even though glasses and braces are not circumferential they present many of the same challenges as bras such as metal, lymph impairment, and restrictive movement of the cranium. With our combined treatment of osteopathy and orthodontia we found patients were finishing treatment earlier. There was a decrease in tooth soreness, patients reported shorter duration, after braces were adjusted.

What other clothing items can we think of that impair lymphatic flow? Shapers, "Spanx," girdles, and socks. Huh? Socks?

Years ago early in my practice, I had a lovely patient in her 70's. Always well-dressed, she arrived in neatly polished low-heeled dress shoes and complementary knee-high hosiery. When she removed the shoes for a treatment her feet and toes stayed in the same shape, as if they had been poured into a mold and dried. I was sure it was from wearing the slender shoes for so many years, it seemed obvious. When I examined her feet I realized it was the springy elastic fibers of the hosiery shaping the foot! The daily application of the elastic tube sock mashed the foot resulting in something like the squished face of a convenience store burglar with pantyhose pulled over their head. Like the evolution of corset to bra I wondered if spandex stockings were an unintended progression of the ancient practice of foot binding in China.

Any sock can be problematic. "Arch support" socks are particularly concerning. Have you seen this design of socks where the mid-section is knitted smaller and elasticized? The tightened area squeezes the mid-foot but lacks the physics to provide lift to the arch. Can you imagine squeezing an inchworm halfway down and telling it this will help it lift its middle? What really happens with a sock like this is a disruption of electrical energy such as nerve impulses and subtle energy such as six of the acupuncture meridians that either begin or end in the toes and forefoot. Echoing the tight bra band dysfunctions, there is disruption of the movement of fluid in the extracellular matrix. There is an allure to the socks, I concede. I recall pulling one on and appreciating the snug fit like a glove. My foot was shaped a little odd but I left it on. Within the hour both feet were cold and there was the light sensation of pins and needles in the forefoot. Socks should feel more like mittens than gloves, I decided.

I've read that fragrances have beginning, middle, and end notes. A perfume that smells divine on first whiff may change mid-stride and end on a sour note when worn. What a great analogy for clothing as well. How does the foot feel pulling on a fresh sock? How does it feel in an hour and at the end of the day? If it is not supporting you comfortably through all these phases, take it off!

It turns out we start early with the spandex sock foot binding.

"What a sweet plump baby! What thighs!" I thought. She will appreciate those when she starts pulling up. But wait, where are her feet? What are those? Little nubbins? I tugged at the little pink sock bands wedged into a skin fold at her ankles. Peeling them off, I found the perfect ten tiny toes twinkling at the end of surprisingly small feet. Compared to the fullness of the ballooned thighs and calves, the feet were deflated, tied off. The tiny elastic socks lie not so innocently nearby.

Do you know why sheep have short tails? They are born with long tails but they are hard to keep clean. The shepherd places a rubber band on the newborn lamb's tail at the desired length. The band squeezes the blood vessels, nerves, and fluids. The tail atrophies and falls off.

Okay, back to the little cutie and her tail, her feet, I mean. Standing on these miniatures would be a challenge. Placing my hands on the feet and legs I sensed the vitality of the tissue dropping off from ankle to feet. Hmmm. My favorites for keeping babies feet warm and protected are the built-in footies of one-piece rompers and pants. Read on for a few tips for grown-ups.

Sock tips summary:

- *Elastic and spandex will try to recoil all day. Be aware of the initial size and shape. Take care to avoid socks that are not shaped like feet such as small mid-section "arch-supports."*
- *Wear the least spandex hose possible. For example, avoid full-length pantyhose if knee-highs will suffice.*
- *Avoid wearing "control-top" garments on a daily basis. Snip vertical relief cuts into the waistband of pantyhose.*
- *Be sure toes have plenty of room to wiggle in hose or socks. Pull them toward the toes a little for room to expand.*
- *If your socks are leaving marks or dents on your leg, they are too tight and inhibiting the flow of circulation. Try folding them down or trimming them to an ankle length.*

Good clothing choice is good self-care. Up next learn ways to move your lymph and care for your breasts and more!

13

Breast Health and Self-care

Energy, movement and lymph drainage

It's the week before your menstrual period and nothing fits, especially the bra. The breasts seem to have doubled in volume and the increase in tenderness is logarithmic! It seems like all a woman can do is wait it out and stock two sizes of clothes. But, lymph is fluid. Fluid is water and water moves fast when it has a way out. We read one story of lymph and swelling in the anatomy section. Another one is the story of a young woman who came to the office for pregnancy discomforts. In addition to rib pain and back ache her lower legs and feet were so swollen she couldn't put on her shoes. She arrived in borrowed fluffy house slippers that still left impressions in her skin. As I gently treated the pelvis and diaphragm then engaged the lower legs directly to free the return pathway for lymph she began to breathe easier. After ten minutes or so, and a trip to the bathroom, we both looked at her feet with astonishment. The tight, smooth skin and sausage-shaped foot had disappeared revealing a slim ankle and individual toes with normal little creases over the joints. She grabbed for the slippers for another fast trip to the potty, but the now floppy fluffies fell off!

Lymphatic congestion cause and effect can form a difficult cycle. Swollen, congested, tender breasts can find temporary relief in tight binding cups that also cause swelling and congestion. Taking little steps such as getting out of underwires, molded cups, and tight bra bands can lead to noticeable changes. In this section we will learn ways to reduce congestion and how to support the movement of lymph through the tissue.

To begin, be sure to hydrate well every day. Drink plenty of clean filtered water, fresh juice, and non-caffeinated tea. Staying hydrated is the first step in improving the quality of the interstitial fluid, the lymph, and will help its ability to circulate and drain.

In her blog, *Nutritious Movement*, Katie Bowman gives creative examples to incorporate movement back into daily tasks in a playful way. We have become a nation of sitters but also of sedentary shoulders. Make use of the built-in lymph equipment by using your arms and shoulders. Pectoralis muscles aren't just for guys. These muscles move fascia, lymph, and blood as well as provide a foundation for the breast.

Now, let's look at a movement routine you can do for yourself to maintain healthy breasts.

The following exercises are most effective when wearing a loose-fitting top without a bra. You can do them anytime though by unhooking and loosening your bra.

A. **Stretch.** Stretch your arms overhead and side to side to open up the underarm area. Take several full breaths in and out.
B. **Dangle.** Lean forward allowing the breasts to lift naturally off the chest wall. Take several relaxing breaths here.
C. **Massage.** Massage or tap the following neurolymphatic points.
- **Spleen and liver**: These are along the imaginary bottom of a bra cup.
- **Lungs**: These are in the crease between the shoulder and chest. It would match up to a sleeve seam in the front.
- **Kidneys**: Slide fingertips just below (inferior to) collarbones on either side of the sternum. There is a little dip or dent there. These points may be tender like some of the other neurolymphatic points.

- **Pericardium**: These points are deep to the nipple close to the chest wall. To reach them use a leaning forward posture. Gently slide the breast tissue of one breast toward your center line until you can reach the rib area that was under the nipple. This is the space between the 4th and 5th ribs. This point is often tender. Gently massage the area then release the breast to its natural position. Repeat on the other side.
D. **Cross-over Energy:** Donna Eden of Energy Medicine describes the effect of shoulder bags on the body's energy pattern. The energy lines are "cut-through" at the arm and shoulder. The same principle applies to bra shoulder straps. To correct this pattern, "cross-overs" can be done to move energy from right to left to re-establish a healthy pattern. The following version I use is inspired by Donna's cross-over as well as my background in dance and osteopathy. An everyday version can be as simple as an exaggerated arm swing while walking.
- Reach over your left shoulder with the right hand. Sweep the hand from left shoulder to right hip. Now repeat with the right shoulder to the left hip. Three cycles with refreshing relaxing breaths are a great start. You can repeat this movement anytime through the day and experience a re-boot of your vitality!

Shared lymph nodes

We can reduce the burden of toxins and debris for lymphatic system. Knowledge of potential lymph toxin loaders will give you the insight needed to weigh choices about what goes in or on your skin.

Underarm skin products

Deodorant and antiperspirant products have ingredient labels. Read them with your fine print glasses and decide if those are ingredients that support your cells. As noted earlier in the match-up, nearly anything put on skin can be absorbed through our skin. If the skin is soft, thin skin with lots of blood vessels and warmth absorption is increased. Open the skin with micro-cuts and abrasions and there is even more absorption. Recall in the anatomy and bra sections that breast tissue extends up toward the armpit and into the armpit in some people. You get the picture.

Underarm products are potentially absorbed directly into breast tissue. I recommend researching some of the many products now available for non-toxic deodorant options. The most common complaint I have heard over the years is that "natural" deodorants smell great until you actually need deodorant. But, the current array seems to have something for everyone without the toxins. The internet is full of recipes for DIY deodorants as well. Many of these use baking soda, clay, or charcoal as a base. These are all very alkaline. Skin is naturally slightly acidic so these recipes need to be buffered to avoid irritation. Trimming underarm hair can help reduce surface area for bacteria and help with odor control.

Antiperspirants are often found in deodorants but are a separate category. Antiperspirants work by creating a gel-like plug in the sweat gland opening with aluminum. This can do double damage, first by putting aluminum on skin and into pores where it is absorbed and second by disabling a natural detoxification mechanism; sweating. What to do? Go retro on this one. Dress-pads are cotton pads that secure to the inside of a shirt to absorb excess perspiration.

Finally, and this is a bit further into the scope of health, really look into what makes you sweat (and smell bad). What stressors, what diet, what parts of your life "stink"?

This first step to preventing smelliness is self-care of the whole person. Feeling safe, breathing, hydrating, good nutrition, and physical activity are basic needs. Support your parasympathetic nervous system with tools such as meditation, mindfulness, and prayer. The parasympathetic nervous system includes the vagus nerve carrying calm "rest and digest" signals to your body and brain. Build on this calm safe state to make fresh positive changes in your lifestyle.

Shaving

I have often wondered about the effect shaving underarms has on lymph nodes. The most obvious observation is skin irritation, red bumps or a rash after shaving that can persist for days, often until the hair is noticeable again and ready for the next shave. Many topical skin products will warn a consumer "Do not use on broken skin." That is precisely what a rash, irritated or cut skin is. And, it's exactly what happens next to freshly shaven underarms; deodorant or antiperspirant is applied to the broken skin. I think of the millions of skin flora; bacteria, fungi, viruses, and debris and now chemicals that just got a free pass to the interstitial fluid. That fluid passes on to lymph vessels to be packaged in lymph nodes, many of them shared with the breast. That's a lot of debris taxing the lymph nodes, our detoxification pathway for breasts. My recommendation for underarm care is rather practical. If you have any sensitivity such as rash or soreness with shaving, consider not shaving! Or consider how often it is necessary. Perhaps trimming the hair close but not abrading the skin will suffice. Maybe it will just be a summertime grooming activity.

Tattoos

It's 3 a.m., and I've just taken my first break in the 12 hour E.R. shift. As I walk down the hall toward a cup of tea that I won't have time to drink, my mind wanders, processing events of the night. Where do tattoos go? Former Marines with naked ladies that danced on their once-toned biceps, floral arrangements on ankles of great aunts...

I mentally fixate on an earlier encounter with a fierce fire-tiger escaping its confines from below the belt.

"That's quite vibrant," I comment.

"Yeah, thanks. It's new," she responded. "It'll fade."

Until then I had innocently thought tattoos must wear off, dulling with time. Nope. It is the magic of the immune and lymphatic cleanup crew doing its job, breaking down foreign substances and sweeping up debris. The proof, it seems, is in the lymph nodes. Multiple studies have shown a rainbow of ink in lymph nodes downstream of tattoos. The breakdown of body art deposits in these drainage nodes. For the arms, chest, and back these nodes are shared with lymph from the breast, which places an additional strain on the maintenance crew.

Light and temperature regulation are two more examples of what goes on and into our bodies.

Light

In chapter 4, Bodies and Bras: The Match-Up, emerging science behind light, photons, and our cells is introduced. Full spectrum light, sunlight, is needed for healthy cells. The amount, measured in strength of light and duration of exposure, is really unknown. And, it would need to be further individualized for each person. Specifically individualized for the amount of melanin, melanopsin in retinal and skin melanophores, rhodopsin in retinal rods, photopsin in retinal cones, age, hydration, and the season. But, we do know that we need light and I suggest a modest amount directly on skin. This could be as little as 5 to 10 minutes of early morning light for a fair complexion, on a regular basis. Light therapies are an area to keep an eye on as information develops. For now, a bit of full spectrum light, avoiding turning even the slightest pink in the sun, staying well-hydrated, avoiding overheating, and avoiding high UV index exposure is sensible. When possible, this means light exposure to the skin of the breasts and underarms, too.

Temperature

I hope this isn't too graphic. But, certain human body parts are loose and not tucked inside the body cavity for a reason. Testicles are a prime example. Toasty testes have a lower sperm count. Their best adaptation is to have their own thermostat. Therefore, they are stationed outside the body cavity in rumpled sacs that have the ability to wrinkle and lift-up or unwrinkle and hang loose. It's ingenious really. Now, I am not saying breasts are analogous to testicles. But, we've all noticed that breasts are also on the outside of the body with access to auto-regulation of temperature. Cold produces lifting and tightening of breasts and heat lets tissue relax and increase surface area to cool. Breasts can't auto-cool if they are inhibited by clothing layers adhered to skin and pressed into the body.

Check the temperature inside a bra while wearing it sometime. Compare it to the temperature of neighboring skin or skin with the bra off for at least 30 minutes.

Hormone production and cellular function changes throughout the menstrual cycle for women. So much so that daily basal temperature readings in tenths of a degree Fahrenheit can help a woman determine what part of the cycle she is in. Humans survive in a narrow range of temperature variation. Our optimal range for cellular function is even smaller, down to the hundredths of a degree we know. How are we affecting cellular function of breast, adipose, and lymph tissue with prolonged heating? What can we do to mitigate it?

Start with natural fibers next to skin such as cotton, linen, silk, or wool. Surprisingly, wool can be soft! I discovered this with baby diaper covers, so soft, no scratchy sensation, and no more diaper rash. These natural fibers regulate temperature better than synthetics. Woven fabrics are less clingy than knits. Knits are capable of being more form-fitting. Whenever possible opt for a loose- fitting piece like a camisole or undershirt for best temperature regulation.

The next section, thermography, summarizes many of the principles of maintaining healthy tissue in a surprising way.

Thermography

Today I am going to try thermography and add the findings to other breast imaging, specifically, mammogram and ultrasound. I am curious to see how it compares and what information it adds. The biggest benefit is that it is completely non-toxic! Thermography is a photograph that images heat. No contact, no radiation. While reading the instructions to prepare for my thermography appointment I was struck with parallels I had been sharing with patients for so long. The list of do's and don'ts for the day of the appointment turned out to look like my bra lecture and self-care recommendations!

Avoid the following for 24 hours prior to your appointment:

- deodorant, antiperspirant, topical essential oils

- shaving underarms
- tight, fitted or clingy clothing (yes, bras)
- hot showers or baths
- bodywork, acupuncture
- smoking or drinking alcohol

Thermography, heat sensing photography, in medicine has been around since the 1950s. In conversation with thermologist, Dr. Leando, I learned that Europe has had a longer history of use and application of thermography in the clinic and hospital. It is frequently used in the emergency department setting there to assess injuries. Thermography creates images from infrared heat radiating from skin. A trained thermographer takes photos using an infrared high-resolution camera. The thermographer uses a specific protocol to ensure standardized images. These images are sent to a thermologist, a physician trained to interpret the images, for a reading. A thermologist can distinguish patterns of injury, acute and chronic infection, chronic sympathetic nervous system hyperactivity, and altered lymph drainage. A thermologist's course of study includes vascular health, musculoskeletal, neurologic, and women's health specialties.

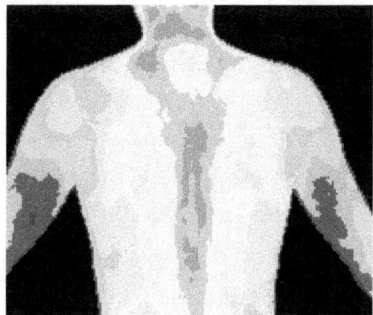

Figure: 13.1: Thermograph of upper back and arms
Light to dark correlates with cool to warm temperatures.

Why was the pre-appointment list made? Because, all of these actions affect the blood flow to and from tissues. They each alter lymph drainage and modify signals in the nervous system. Each of these modifications can be seen as temperature patterns on our skin. If the thermography interpretation can be changed by these daily activities, what are these activities doing to us over time?

Although we may not have given much thought until now to getting dressed, shaving underarms, putting on deodorant and bras we can be mindful of these choices. If the camera can see the body's response in a photo what does our body experience on a cellular level? Changes in blood circulation and lymph flow, compression of organs, muscle, and bone day after day have an effect on overall health. And, we have a choice!

14

Bras, Breasts, and Beyond: Engaging the Breast Appreciation Group

In *Breasts: A Natural and Unnatural History,* author Florence Williams interviews a pair of male researchers studying what features men first notice about women and what keeps their attention. It seems that men were attracted to just about anything on the female, but specifically female traits ranked higher, like breasts with nipples. The attraction may be hard-wired just like the desire to provide protection.

In general, men are fascinated by bras and the breasts that lie beneath them. The idea of the bra not being there and just the "under" part seems to be the prevailing thought pattern. When hearing the possibility of a bra causing deformity of ribs and organs, men are alert and concerned; both in regard to "Why didn't I think of that?" and deep concern over the well-being of their loved-ones. A man on a mission to provide protection is a valuable ally.

Mr. Fix-It hats went on when veils of illusion were lifted and emotions peaked.

"What? Those backless, strapless celebrity gowns are held up by foam cups and duct tape?! "

"Padding and push-up? Hey! That's false advertising!"

"I get it, I pulled a tiny sports bra out of the dryer and thought my baby girl was growing up. My wife grabbed it and put in her drawer with a nest of other ones! I was relieved but wondered, 'How?'"

These reactions quickly shifted into solution mode. Engineering plans flew through the air in a verbal banter. I wish I could say we designed the perfect solution, a hydraulic lacey lift allowing lymphatic drainage. We realized the perfect solution is not just one design. The wonderful variety of women and their myriad of activities require a wonderful variety of solutions. I mean, really, can one pair of shoes excel at everything? Sometimes it's good to be barefoot.

In recent times, the move toward working from home opened the door to new wardrobe options. A friend said that after we had talked about the effects of bras, she questioned why she was wearing one at home. So she took it off. She wondered what her husband would think. Would he be uncomfortable? Would he even notice? A smile lifted her brow when she confided weeks later, "He seems pretty happy!"

Appendix

Shopping Websites

Although "it's always a compromise" per my dear friend, here are some sites that can satisfy a goal or two.

Brastop (https://us.brastop.com/): Brastop shows a selection of medium to full cup and band sizes.

The Little Bra Company (https://www.thelittlebracompany.com/): These selections range in the medium to petite cup sizes and smaller bands.

Title Nine (https://www.titlenine.com/): Title Nine features sports bras for many body shapes and athletic adventures. Remember to only wear chest compression for brief periods of time! Look for a high neckline in front and back closures that can be released or adjusted.

Vibrant (https://vibrantbodycompany.com): A selection of bras made from non-toxic materials, wire-free anatomical cups, cotton blend, and silk blend undergarments.

True & Co. (https://trueandco.com/): The True Body line offers multiple wire-free styles. Consider sizing up by 2 for better ribcage motion.

The following links are based on fiber, not fit. The few I reviewed were still a fit challenge for bras and panties. Remember to ignore the size guideline charts and ask for the actual garment dimensions. The following have organic, natural fibers or upcycled, recycled, and eco-friendly options:

Boody (https://boodywear.com/): An Australian company providing men's and women's underlayers and socks of bamboo viscose.

Icebreaker (https://www.icebreaker.com/): Merino wool first layers for men and women from an outdoor adventure company.

Princesse Tam.Tam (https://www.princessetamtam.com/): Glamorous designs with some Oeko-Tex 100 options are shown here.

Pact (https://wearpact.com/): Organic cotton skivvies for men and women.

Reformation (https://www.thereformation.com/): Eco-friendly recycled and up-cycled fibers are featured. (Not necessarily low toxins)

Wama Underwear (https://wamaunderwear.com/) Wama features organic hemp first layers.

Woron (https://www.woronstore.com/): Woron's site has curated bras of low to no toxins in Oeko-Tex 100 fabrics.

References and Resources

Anatomy Visualized 3-D
Alexander Tsiarias and Barry Werth. 2004 The Architecture and Design of Man and Woman, Doubleday division of Random House
Anti-perspirant
Darbre P. D. (2016). Aluminium and the human breast. *Morphologie : bulletin de l'Association des anatomistes*, *100*(329), 65–74. https://doi.org/10.1016/j.morpho.2016.02.001
Mannello, F., Tonti, G. A., & Darbre, P. D. (2009). Concentration of aluminum in breast cyst fluids collected from women affected by gross cystic breast disease. *Journal of applied toxicology : JAT*, *29*(1), 1–6. https://doi.org/10.1002/jat.1384
Bra-fitting
Cudby, Ali. 2017. Fit My Bras, How to Find Your Perfect Bra and Why it Matters, 2cnd edition. CreateSpace Independent Publishing Platform
Luciani, Jene. 2017. The Bra Book, An intimate Guide to Finding the Right Bra, Shapewear, Swimsuit and More! BenBella Books.
Bra Sizing, Design and Materials
Lehman, Heidi. 2020. In discussion with the author. The Vibrant Bra Company, https://vibrantbodycompany.com/
Tempesta, Laura. (Feb 7, 2019). You'll never look at a bra the same way again. TedxKC. https://www.youtube.com/watch?v=GrxJ-9_qXeM
Electrical and EMF
Becker, Robert. 1998 The Body Electric, William Morrow Paperbacks
Chockattu, S. J., Suryakant, D. B., & Thakur, S. (2018). Unwanted effects due to interactions between dental materials and magnetic resonance imaging: a review of the literature. *Restorative dentistry & endodontics*, *43*(4), e39. https://doi.org/10.5395/rde.2018.43.e39
Hasegawa, M., Miyata, K., Abe, Y., & Ishigami, T. (2013). Radiofrequency heating of metallic dental devices during 3.0 T MRI. *Dento maxillo facial radiology*, *42*(5), 20120234. https://doi.org/10.1259/dmfr.20120234
Mortazavi, S., Dehghani Nazhvani, A., & Paknahad, M. (2019). Synergistic Effect of Radiofrequency Electromagnetic Fields of Dental Light Cure Devices and

Mobile Phones Accelerates the Microleakage of Amalgam Restorations: An in vitro Study. *Journal of biomedical physics & engineering, 9*(2), 227–232.

Ryan Blaser, 2021. Building Biology- https://testmyhome.com. In communication with the author.

Energy Medicine

Dale, Cyndi. 2009. The Subtle Body: An Encyclopedia of Your Energetic Anatomy. Sounds True, Inc. Boulder, CO

Eden, Donna. 2008. Energy Medicine, 2nd Edition. (Feinstein, D., Myss, C., Gartner, ?.) Jeremy P. Tarcher

Light Therapy

Alves, A. N., Fernandes, K. P., Deana, A. M., Bussadori, S. K., & Mesquita-Ferrari, R. A. (2014). Effects of low-level laser therapy on skeletal muscle repair: a systematic review. *American journal of physical medicine & rehabilitation, 93*(12), 1073–1085. https://doi.org/10.1097/PHM.0000000000000158

Huang YY, Gupta A, Vecchio D, et al. Transcranial low level laser (light) therapy for traumatic brain injury. J Biophotonics. 2012;5(11-12):827-837. doi:10.1002/jbio.201200077

Kazem Shakouri, S., Soleimanpour, J., Salekzamani, Y., & Oskuie, M. R. (2010). Effect of low-level laser therapy on the fracture healing process. *Lasers in medical science, 25*(1), 73–77. https://doi.org/10.1007/s10103-009-0670-7

Sutherland J. C. (2002). Biological effects of polychromatic light. *Photochemistry and photobiology, 76*(2), 164–170. https://doi.org/10.1562/0031-8655(2002)0760164BEOPL2.0.CO2

Xuan, W., Vatansever, F., Huang, L., Wu, Q., Xuan, Y., Dai, T., Ando, T., Xu, T., Huang, Y. Y., & Hamblin, M. R. (2013). Transcranial low-level laser therapy improves neurological performance in traumatic brain injury in mice: effect of treatment repetition regimen. *PloS one, 8*(1), e53454. https://doi.org/10.1371/journal.pone.0053454

Lymphatics Osteopathic

Chapman, Frank. 1983. An Endocrine Interpretation of Chapman's Reflexes. American Academy of Osteopathy, Indianapolis, IN

Chikly, Bruno. 2017. Silent Waves, Theory and Practice of lymph Drainage Therapy. 3rd edition. Chikly Health Institite,

Lymph and Tattoos

Sepehri, M., Sejersen, T., Qvortrup, K., Lerche, C. M., & Serup, J. (2017). Tattoo Pigments Are Observed in the Kupffer Cells of the Liver Indicating Blood-Borne Distribution of Tattoo Ink. *Dermatology (Basel, Switzerland), 233*(1), 86–93. https://doi.org/10.1159/000468149

Schreiver, I., Hesse, B., Seim, C., Castillo-Michel, H., Anklamm, L., Villanova, J., Dreiack, N., Lagrange, A., Penning, R., De Cuyper, C., Tucoulou, R., Bäumler, W., Cotte, M., & Luch, A. (2019). Distribution of nickel and chromium containing particles from tattoo needle wear in humans and its possible impact on allergic reactions. *Particle and fibre toxicology, 16*(1), 33. https://doi.org/10.1186/

s12989-019-0317-1Am J Dermatopathol. 2018 May;40(5):383-385. doi: 10.1097/DAD.0000000000001043

Soran, A., Menekse, E., Kanbour-Shakir, A., Tane, K., Diego, E., Bonaventura, M., & Johnson, R. (2017). The importance of tattoo pigment in sentinel lymph nodes. *Breast disease, 37*(2), 73–76. https://doi.org/10.3233/BD-170282

Tamura, D., Maeda, D., Terada, Y., & Goto, A. (2019). Distribution of Tattoo Pigment in Lymph Nodes Dissected for Gynecological Malignancy. *International journal of surgical pathology, 27*(7), 773–777. https://doi.org/10.1177/1066896919846395

Microbiome

Urban J, Fergus DJ, Savage AM, Ehlers M, Menninger HL, Dunn RR, Horvath JE. 2016. The effect of habitual and experimental antiperspirant and deodorant product use on the armpit microbiome. PeerJ 4:e1605 https://doi.org/10.7717/peerj.1605

Movement

Bowman, Katy. https://www.nutritiousmovement.com/blog/

Physiology, Pressure, Mechanics

Lee, Y. A., Hyun, K. J., & Tokura, H. (2000). The effects of skin pressure by clothing on circadian rhythms of core temperature and salivary melatonin. *Chronobiology international, 17*(6), 783–793. https://doi.org/10.1081/cbi-100102114

Lee, Y. A., Kikufuji, N., & Tokura, H. (2000). Field studies on inhibitory influence of skin pressure exerted by a body compensatory brassiere on the amount of feces. *Journal of physiological anthropology and applied human science, 19*(4), 191–194. https://doi.org/10.2114/jpa.19.191

Miyatsuji, A., Matsumoto, T., Mitarai, S., Kotabe, T., Takeshima, T., & Watanuki, S. (2002). Effects of clothing pressure caused by different types of brassieres on autonomic nervous system activity evaluated by heart rate variability power spectral analysis. *Journal of physiological anthropology and applied human science, 21*(1), 67–74. https://doi.org/10.2114/jpa.21.67

Ochs, M., Nyengaard, J. R., Jung, A., Knudsen, L., Voigt, M., Wahlers, T., Richter, J., & Gundersen, H. J. (2004). The number of alveoli in the human lung. *American journal of respiratory and critical care medicine, 169*(1), 120–124. https://doi.org/10.1164/rccm.200308-1107OC

Takasu, N., Furuoka, S., Inatsugi, N., Rutkowska, D., & Tokura, H. (2000). The effects of skin pressure by clothing on whole gut transit time and amount of feces. *Journal of physiological anthropology and applied human science, 19*(3), 151–156. https://doi.org/10.2114/jpa.19.151

Shape shifting

Ashizawa, K., Sugane, A., & Gunji, T. (1990). Breast form changes resulting from a certain brassière. *Journal of human ergology, 19*(1), 53–62.

Transdermal absorption

Atlan, M., & Neman, J. (2019). Targeted Transdermal Delivery of Curcumin for

Breast Cancer Prevention. *International journal of environmental research and public health*, *16*(24), 4949. https://doi.org/10.3390/ijerph16244949

Dave, K., Alsharif, F. M., Islam, S., Dwivedi, C., & Perumal, O. (2017). Chemoprevention of Breast Cancer by Transdermal Delivery of α-Santalol through Breast Skin and Mammary Papilla (Nipple). *Pharmaceutical research*, *34*(9), 1897–1907. https://doi.org/10.1007/s11095-017-2198-z

Drescher, Michael. (2019). Theories on breast cancer. TedxUWMilwaukee, https://www.youtube.com/watch?v=HISv4FgMzYc

Hashimoto, N., Nakamichi, N., Yamazaki, E., Oikawa, M., Masuo, Y., Schinkel, A. H., & Kato, Y. (2017). P-Glycoprotein in skin contributes to transdermal absorption of topical corticosteroids. *International journal of pharmaceutics*, *521*(1-2), 365–373. https://doi.org/10.1016/j.ijpharm.2017.02.064

Lee, O., & Khan, S. A. (2016). Novel routes for administering chemoprevention: local transdermal therapy to the breasts. *Seminars in oncology*, *43*(1), 107–115. https://doi.org/10.1053/j.seminoncol.2015.09.003

Acknowledgements

I offer a heartfelt thank you to all who contributed to the production of Booby Traps; A Book of Bras, Breasts, and Bands. They include, but are not limited to:

My patients of 30 years who inspired me to look further and teach more often, newly minted book coach, Starlight Katsaros, who wears many hats well, and my writing group; Deb, Leslie, and Marcella. Thank you also to physician and writer, Dave Walker, M.D. (*God in the ICU*) for timely words of encouragement and physician and writer, Arlene Dijamco, M.D. (I AM Intuitive - A MultiDimensional Guide to Embrace Your Inner Light) for multidimensional clarity. More gratitude goes to manuscript reading, editing, and art critique; Jenn, Jennifer Grace, Artie, Monica, Lisa Brice, MSW, LCSW, Holly Amjad, David Spencer, D.O., and Laurie Connolly Braun. Research support came from Truman State University librarian Annie Moots and A.T. Still University, Laura Lipke, MS, MLIS, AHIP. Digital art solutions were gracefully assisted by Katie Johnson and Natalie Montefinese. Publishing guidance was gratefully accepted by authors Artie Lynnworth, John Burley, M.D., and Toni Rahman, LCSW.

Special thanks to my husband, David, and our family. Thank you to our parents, my brother, our sisters, aunts, uncles, cousins, kiddos, and grandkids. You have played the biggest role in support of this book production.

About the Author

A 1995 graduate of Kirksville College of Osteopathic Medicine, Dr. Coffman has experienced an osteopathic medical career that resembles a jungle hike through the mountains emerging on clear, sparkling shores. Her early career focused on emergency medicine and further developed her resourceful nature and acute care skills. In 2001, she founded Hands On Health Osteopathic Medicine and began to treat the chronic effects of injury and illness while continuing to transform the practice to include prevention of both acute and chronic health concerns. Careful to incorporate intuition into every step, Dr. Coffman accepted the notion to write and illustrate for others what she has been treating and teaching for several decades.

As a mom of 3, she loves keeping up with one very fast teen, two self-sufficient young adults, and energy-filled grandchildren. She and her husband, David, live in Missouri where they nibble wild plums and other tasty things.

She relaxes with art, acroyoga, grandchildren, and being in nature, preferably all at the same time.

www.ingramcontent.com/pod-product-compliance
Lightning Source LLC
LaVergne TN
LVHW020438070526
838199LV00063B/4774